FROM BENCH TO BEDSIDE - TRAUMA, TUMORS, SPINE, FUNCTIONAL NEUROSURGERY

Edited by **Francesco Signorelli**

From Bench to Bedside - Trauma, Tumors, Spine, Functional Neurosurgery
http://dx.doi.org/10.5772/61624
Edited by Francesco Signorelli

Contributors

Sergio D Bergese, Juan Fiorda-Diaz, Nicoleta Stoicea, Milind Deogaonkar, Luiz Claudio Rodrigues, Massimo Miscusi, Alessandro Pesce, Antonino Raco, Hae Yu Kim, Linda Papa, Kimberly Rosenthal, Alba Scerrati, Mario Ammirati, Lijun Ma, Dilini Pinnaduwage, Peng Dong, Giuseppe Messina, Massimo Leone, Angelo Franzini, Alberto Proietti Cecchini

Published by InTech

Janeza Trdine 9, 51000 Rijeka, Croatia

Publishing Process Manager Andrea Koric

Technical Editor SPi Global

Cover InTech Design team

First published October, 2016

Printed in Croatia

Additional hard copies can be obtained from orders@intechopen.com

From Bench to Bedside - Trauma, Tumors, Spine, Functional Neurosurgery, Edited by Francesco Signorelli

p. cm.

Print ISBN 978-953-51-2628-7
Online ISBN 978-953-51-2629-4

For EU product safety concerns:
IN TECH d.o.o., Prolaz Marije Krucifikse Kozulić 3, 51000 Rijeka, Croatia,
info@intechopen.com or visit our website at intechopen.com.

Meet the editor

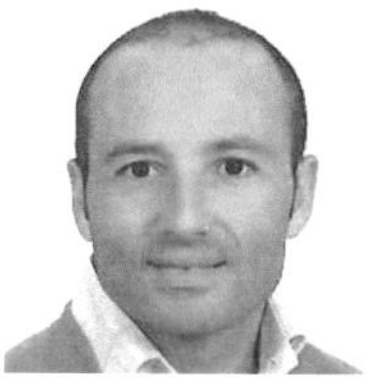

Professor Francesco Signorelli is an Italian board-certified neurosurgeon. He completed his neurosurgery training at the University Hospital of Naples, Italy, and fellow in neurosurgery in London and Southampton, UK, and fellow in vascular neurosurgery and skull base neurosurgery at the University Hospital in Montreal, Canada. He worked as an associate professor of neurosurgery at the University Hospital of Catanzaro, Italy, and more recently he has rejoined the staff of the "P. Wertheimer" Hospital for Neurology and Neurosurgery in Lyon, France. His surgical practice has canvassed the spectrum of neurosurgery together with his scientific activity, with over 3000 interventions, more than 50 articles in peer-reviewed journals, and several book chapters and review articles. He is a member of national and international neurosurgical associations and of the French humanitarian association "Association pour le Développement Médical au Vietnam." His current major interests are vascular neurosurgery, skull base surgery, and surgery of brain tumors in eloquent areas.

Contents

Preface

Neurosurgeons should have a fundamental knowledge of the scientific evidence regarding all pathologies they confronted with. Such knowledge can lead to a high level of expertise and properly guide patients' management. This book was conceived as an example of the aforementioned integrated approach to some of the commonest pathologies a neurosurgeon deals with on a daily basis. The aim of the book is not completeness, but rather it dives into selected main subjects of neurosurgery, from head trauma to deep brain stimulation, dealing with open surgical and radiosurgical techniques for brain and spine tumors. The authors of the eight chapters are outstanding researchers and clinicians devoted to the spreading of their knowledge through this open source book, which hopefully will reach the widespread diffusion of the two other books that preceded the current one. This book is written for graduate students, researchers, and practitioners who are interested in learning how the knowledge from research can be implemented in clinical competences. The first section is dedicated to deep brain stimulation, a surgical procedure which is the paramount example of how clinical practice can take advantage from fundamental research. The second section gathers five chapters and illustrates how significant is the challenge to translate scientific advances into clinical practice because the route from evidence to action is not always obvious. It is hoped that this book will stimulate the interest in the process of translating research into practice for a broader range of neurosurgical topics than the one covered by this book, which could result in a forthcoming more comprehensive publication.

I wish to thank all authors for their excellent contribution to the book; without their enthusiastic participation, this book project would have not been possible. Finally, I thank Ms. Andrea Koric, the InTech publishing process manager, whose competence and kind patience in stimulating all participants, including myself, were invaluable in finalizing this book. I am especially grateful to my wife Vanessa and my daughter Alice for their understanding and support, so that I could spend many extra hours working on this book.

Francesco Signorelli, MD, MSc
Consultant Neurosurgeon, Hospices Civils de Lyon, France
Associate Professor of Neurosurgery, University "Magna Græcia," Catanzaro, Italy

Section 1

From Basic Neuroscience to Treatment: Deep Brain Stimulation

Chapter 1

Anesthetic Considerations for Deep Brain Stimulation

Juan Fiorda-Diaz, Nicoleta Stoicea,
Milind S. Deogaonkar and Sergio D. Bergese

Additional information is available at the end of the chapter

http://dx.doi.org/10.5772/63984

Abstract

Deep brain stimulation (DBS) was used to treat refractory Parkinson's disease (PD) for the first time in 1987 by Professor Benabid's group by placing stimulating electrodes into targeted brain structures. DBS is a widely accepted neurosurgical treatment for Parkinson's disease (PD), benign tremor, dystonia, epilepsy, and other neuropsychiatric disorders with no significant changes in anatomical brain structures. Prior to the introduction of DBS, traditional treatment for PD involved surgical removal of parts of the brain known as thalamotomy, pallidotomy, and cingulotomy. Intraoperative identification of the affected areas of brain is possible through a couple of mechanisms involving electrical stimulation and monitoring of the brain function, known as "functional neurosurgery". Implantation of electrodes in the targeted area and the insertion of a programmable pulse generator under the clavicle or in the abdomen are the main steps in DBS surgery. Anesthetic management for DBS remains controversial and might vary between institutions and physicians. Although no guidelines have been developed, there are some common anesthetic considerations for DBS surgery, including difficult airway management, facilitation of neuromonitoring, and anesthetic drugs interference with microelectrode recordings (MERs). Local anesthesia, general anesthesia, and monitored anesthesia care (MAC) have been used worldwide in patients undergoing DBS.

Keywords: deep brain stimulation, functional neurosurgery, neurodegenerative disorders, general anesthesia, monitored care anesthesia

1. Introduction

1.1. Technique and physiological considerations

Imaging techniques play an essential role in neurological diseases, offering precise information of anatomical location of the lesion, facilitating the identification, description, and prognostic evaluation of the disease in the vast majority of cases.

Affected areas of brain, contributing to patient signs and symptoms, may vary according to the type of disorder and treatment. Therapeutic protocols have been elaborated based on signs and symptoms, and different patient response. Modern medicine offers intraoperative identification of affected areas through a couple of mechanisms involving electrical stimulation and intraoperative brain function monitoring, known as "functional neurosurgery" [1].

Deep brain stimulation (DBS) is known as a neurosurgical treatment for several functional disorders through neuromodulation. Its use has been described in Parkinson's disease (PD), benign tremor, dystonia, epilepsy, and psychiatric disorders with no significant changes in anatomical brain structures [2].

Molecular and physiological responses to DBS are deeply studied. Several mechanisms have been described, including inhibition and stimulation processes that induce different reactions, not only in the targeted area but also in its vicinity [3]. Velasco et al. showed some variations in metabolism of five patients with PD after DBS of prelemniscal radiations (RAPRL), using F-FDG PET (2-deoxy-2-fluoro-D-glucose positron emission tomography). In order to corroborate definitive electrodes' position, microelectrode recordings (MERs) and macrostimulation were performed during the insertion process. They concluded that DBS produces a significant clinical improvement in these patients as a result of the reduction in metabolic rate in the Raprl, which led to decreased electrical responses of these cells in spite of high stimulation rates [4].

Characteristics of the stimulus are dependent on some modifiable factors such as type (monopolar or bipolar), frequency (usually high-frequency ranges), amplitude, and pulse width [5]. With respect to the physiological basis of neurons' connections, monosynaptic and polysynaptic functioning should be taken into consideration. Therefore, identification of dysfunctional areas and their networks in terms of derived extensive signaling would categorize eligibility of patients for DBS treatment [5] as well as the most suitable anesthesia technique for each case.

Implantation of electrodes in the targeted area and the insertion of a programmable pulse generator under the clavicle or in the abdomen are the main steps in DBS surgery [1, 6]. Generators might work during a few years, depending on the stimulation rates, although some of them are rechargeable [5]. The process of electrodes' placement is guided by MERs and concomitant macrostimulation, which consists of intraoperative physical stimulus or mental tasks to assess the responses of patients to DBS [7]. Anesthetic drugs have an important impact at this stage of the surgery [7, 8].

Surgery-related complications include perioperative and hardware-related issues. Beric et al. published in 2001 their experience with 86 patients and 149 DBS surgeries. They described perioperative complications in eight patients (hemorrhages, confusion, and seizures) and long-term postoperative complications in eight patients (delayed hematoma, behavioral changes, confusion, apraxia of eyelid opening, and peripheral nerve injury). Hardware-related issues were studied in nine patients (DBS electrode failure, extension wire failure, pulse generator malfunction, and pain over pulse generator) and stimulation-induced side effects were diagnosed in four patients (dysarthria, facial contraction, and confusion) [9].

2. Deep brain stimulation: history

2.1. DBS history

Electrical stimulation of an affected zone by placing an "electric fish" on its surface was surprisingly used from ancient eras up to eighteenth century. Headaches, epilepsy, and gout benefit of its clinical use [2, 10].

In the last century, DBS surgery was associated with three major events. In 1947, the use of a stereotactic device in humans was first described as "stereoencephalotomy" [11]. In 1952, local low-frequency stimulation was implemented in psychiatric interventions, leading to a successful use of high-frequency stimulation in patients with intractable tremor in 1987 [11, 12]. In 1997, Food and Drug Administration (FDA) approved the use of DBS in patients with essential tremor (ET) [2].

Prior to the introduction of DBS, the stereotactic frame was commonly used in surgical removal of parts of the brain, such as thalamotomy, pallidotomy, and cingulotomy in patients with functional pathologies. From this point on, the use of ablation techniques led to several clinical responses obtained from stimulation at low frequency and high frequency, with relevant findings in patients with Parkinson's disease [13]. Nevertheless, the introduction of levodopa during the 1960s offset existing interest in stereotactic surgery [14].

In 1991, Benabid et al. published data from 32 patients diagnosed with levodopa-resistant tremor, 18 of them with past surgical history of bilateral thalamic surgery. Electrodes and semi-microelectrodes were used to stimulate ventral intermediate nucleus (VIM) with high frequency (100 Hz or more), being stimulation-adjusted depending on the level of tremor suppression. After definitive placement of electrodes, general anesthesia (GA) was administered to insert a programmable stimulator in the chest wall. They concluded that the capability to modify the intensity of the stimulus and other characteristics of this kind of stimulation, such as reversibility of the effects, might have a huge advantage, when compared with thalamotomy [12].

During the last decades, advances in electrophysiology and imaging have allowed more accurate localization of particular altered areas, as well as their different reactions under stimulation, either activation or inhibition, with the consequent widespread of signals [3, 15].

Outcomes in DBS surgery rely on accuracy during the electrodes' insertion and placement. "Indirect" and "direct" techniques describe neuroimaging use during different stages of the procedure [16]. Indirect techniques, involving the use of MERs and a stereotactic frame to identify the targeted area, have been replaced in the vast majority by magnetic resonance imaging (MRI) for direct evaluation of anatomical structures during surgery [16, 17]. Nevertheless, safety MRI use in DBS surgeries follows the current FDA recommendations requiring system integrity [17].

2.2. DBS ethical nuances

As a consequence of satisfactory results obtained from the use of DBS in PD and other movement disorders, interest in showing efficacy of DBS in other disorders such as obesity and obsessive–compulsive disorder among other psychiatric pathologies has been growing in the last decade [18]. Despite the published data from several clinical trials, it is vital to understand that patients' and caregivers' high expectances may be deleterious, mostly in psychiatric patients, as DBS outcomes vary between patients and pathologies. Therefore, ethical issues, such as identifying suitable subjects and their allocation, either in control or in interventional arms, should be considered when designing protocols, to assure patients' safety [18, 19].

Ethical and regulatory committees worldwide should be actively involved in protocols' design regarding DBS surgery in neuropsychiatric patients, emphasizing in all the stages of subjects' participation such as informed consent and misunderstanding of expectations during research [20].

3. Deep brain stimulation: principles and practices

In order to understand the impact of anesthetic drugs either during surgery or in patients' outcomes, it is important to summarize some clinical evidence and to identify the most common targeted structures.

3.1. DBS in movement disorders

Benabid et al. described for the first time in 1987 the use of high-frequency stimulation (100 Hz) in patients with PD. The targeted thalamic nucleus was the ventralis intermedius (VIM), providing an important reduction in bilateral tremor under constant stimulation [21]. Definitely, these outcomes would generate several studies using DBS in patients with movement disorders. The same author published in 1991 a series of 32 patients with intractable tremor who underwent DBS surgery with similar findings. At this time, the authors stated that satisfactory outcomes obtained from continuous VIM stimulation were comparable with those achieved after thalamotomy, suggesting the need for developing new devices that might increase the frequency of stimulation above 100 Hz [12]. Subthalamic nucleus (STN) and globus pallidus interna (GPi) have been described as additional targets for patients with PD, with comparable long-term effects [22].

The ability of DBS to improve quality of life in patients with PD led to its use in different clinical entities, such as hyperkinetic disorders. Montgomery published in 2004 an overview describing patient selection issues generated by these types of disorders, offering a brief description of the pathophysiological aspects and encouraging results of DBS use in this patient population [23].

3.2. DBS in neuropathic pain

Based on previous clinical evidence, Boccard et al. prospectively studied within 12 years, 197 patients diagnosed with neuropathic pain. After excluding patients for several reasons (e.g., contraindications or refusal of surgery), 85 patients were scheduled to undergo DBS surgery. The study was focused on periventricular gray (PVG) area, ventral posterior lateral (VPL), and ventral posterior medial (VPM) thalamic nuclei. Intraoperative macrostimulation was performed instead of MERs to define electrodes' location, and low-frequency (≤50 Hz) stimulations were used with satisfactory results. The procedure was completed with the insertion of the generator in just 74 patients, of which 15 patients did not offer complete data. The authors concluded that despite different degrees of neuropathic pain, the study offers long-term positive responses to DBS [24].

3.3. DBS in neurodegenerative disorders

Recent clinical trials investigated the outcomes of patients diagnosed with moderate dementia of Alzheimer's type scheduled to undergo DBS surgery. The fornix/hypothalamus has been pointed out as the target area of intervention. Laxton et al. published in 2010 a phase I trial, where six patients with Alzheimer's disease (AD) were scheduled for DBS surgery, targeting the fornix/hypothalamus region. Findings were encouraging, with consistent clinical improvement and lesser cognitive decline during 12 months of stimulation [25]. Changes in volumetric measurements of the hippocampus after fornix DBS have also been associated with clinical improvement, suggesting a potential ability of DBS to interfere with the natural progression of the brain atrophy in patients with AD [26]. DBS at variable frequencies and amplitudes has been used with promising results in cognitive impaired animal models [27].

3.4. DBS in psychiatry

Psychiatric disorders are well known as one of the major causes of disability worldwide, depression being the most common among them in both genders, with an annual incidence of 10% of the general population. Between 60 and 70% of patients will experience an improvement, using current antidepressant therapies. Nevertheless, there are an important number of patients where current pharmacology therapies will not lead to satisfactory results [28]. DBS has been shown to be an alternative in these treatment-resistant patients. **Table 1** summarizes most common psychiatric disorders and their areas of interest for DBS [29].

Different areas have been targeted under DBS with satisfactory results in patients with treatment-resistant depression. Lozano et al. studied the outcomes of 20 patients classified within major depressive disorder who underwent subcallosal cingulate gyrus (SCG) DBS. Patients with a decrease in 50% or more in the 17-item Hamilton Rating Scale for Depression (HRSD-17) were considered as "response". They found satisfactory results after 1 week, with

40% of subjects reaching significant reductions in the HRSD-17. Additionally, 60% of subjects reflected significant improvement within the first semester after surgery, whereas 35% reached remission [14].

Target/disease	Depression	Anorexia	OCD	Addiction	Tourette syndrome
Lateral habenula	X				
Subcallosal cingulated	X	X			
Ventral capsule/ventral striatum	X		X	X	
Nucleus accumbens				X	
Inferior thalamic peduncle	X		X		
CM–PF of thalamus					X
GPi/GPe					X
Subthalamic nucleus			X		
Medial forebrain bundle	X				

CM–PF, centromedian–parafascicular nuclear complex; GPi/GPe, globus pallidus (internal/external). Adapted from Cleary et al. [29].

Table 1. DBS and psychiatric disorders: common nuclei for stimulation according to diagnosis.

Despite satisfactory outcomes obtained from clinical trials regarding DBS use in neuropsychiatric patients, it is noticed by the consensus published in 2014 that DBS surgery for any kind of psychiatric disorder has been established as an investigational procedure [20]. With this respect, Hamani et al. carried out an extensive review regarding the uses of DBS in patients with obsessive–compulsive disorder (OCD), concluding that more clinical trials are needed to collect quality evidence before making any recommendations for the therapeutic uses of DBS in this clinical setting, encouraging researchers to develop new protocols in the near future [30].

3.5. DBS in metabolic disorders

Obesity is well known as a public health problem. Recently, Fryar et al. published results from the National Health and Nutrition Examination Survey, concluding that more than two-thirds of the U.S. population is overweight, obese, or extremely obese [31]. Based on the neurohormonal components involving obesity and other metabolic disorders, the questioning of the potential effects of DBS in these patients has emerged.

Hypothalamic stimulation in patients with PD showed potential benefits for obesity as a secondary outcome [32]. Cortico-striato-pallido-thalamo-cortical (CSPTC) circuit activity is associated with obesity. Therefore, stimulation at different sites such as ventromedial hypothalamus and nucleus accumbens might be necessary to obtain satisfactory outcomes [33].

http://dx.doi.org/10.5772/63984

4. Anesthetic considerations in patients undergoing DBS

Currently, limited data has been published with regards to the anesthetic management of DBS with no strict guidelines to follow by healthcare providers [8]. Nevertheless, there are some common concerns for DBS surgery, including patient comfort, Airway and blood pressure management , neuromonitoring, and anesthetic drugs interference with MERs. Particularities of anesthetic management for DBS surgeries with respect to different techniques, their outcomes, and anesthetic-related complications will be discussed.

Local anesthesia (LA), general anesthesia (GA), and monitored anesthesia care (MAC) have been used worldwide in patients undergoing DBS. Advantages and disadvantages have been described for each technique.

Abosch et al. published in 2012 the results of an international survey carried out in 185 DBS centers [34]. All of them were classified based on the number of DBS surgeries per year (1–12 per year, 13–24 per year, 25–52 per year, and >52 per year). Additionally, other variables were studied, such as surgical technique and time of surgery. The primary aim was to identify global factors surrounding DBS surgery, allowing all centers to compare their own experience and to recognize possible difficulties among their counterparts. Local anesthesia was used in 100% of the cases in centers with the lowest number of DBS surgeries per year (1–12 per year), whereas in centers with more than 52 cases per year, only 74% of the patients received local anesthesia, and 26% received general anesthesia. Regarding the type of disorder in patients, 93% of PD patients, 100% of ET patients, and 44% patients with dystonia underwent DBS surgery under local anesthesia [34].

Two main tendencies are noticed regarding the use of LA or GA during DBS surgery. The first one agrees with no use of any systemic anesthetic drug to obtain ideal MERs. Clinical evidence promotes the capabilities of imaging (MRI or MR/CT) to target STN without performing MERs, regardless of the type of anesthesia [35].

Chakrabarti et al. summarized anesthesia management during DBS surgery in three groups, based on patient considerations, surgical techniques, and disease-related [6].

A multidisciplinary preoperative approach is necessary to evaluate the risks of DBS surgery. As neurosurgeons carefully select patients who might benefit from DBS treatment based on certain medical criteria, anesthesiologists are expected to decide the type of anesthesia in a similar manner [36].

4.1. Local Anesthesia

LA as a subcutaneous infiltration or scalp block with long-lasting local anesthetics such as bupivacaine (0.5%), levobupivacaine (0.5%), and ropivacaine (0.75%), potentially offers certain benefits [7]. The absence of interference with MERs, decreased incidence of sedation-related complications such as nausea and vomiting, and reduced effects on hemodynamics or cognitive status are some of the benefits associated with LA.

Different techniques have been described by using LA in patients undergoing neurosurgical procedures, and have been named according to patients' level of consciousness during the stages of the intervention. The awake technique consists of performing scalp block with long–lasting local anesthetics, allowing simultaneous communication between the care team and the patient. This "therapeutic communication" is crucial and may be supplemented with music and other hypnotic techniques during neurosurgery [37].

Combined techniques limiting local anesthetic infiltration to the location of the pins with concomitant conscious sedation, have been described as "asleep-awake-asleep technique". Lange et al reviewed 38 subjects with PD who underwent DBS surgery using two different kind of anesthesia management. Local infiltration with conscious sedation was used in the first group (16 patients), whereas the second group (22 patients) received scalp nerve blockade with any or very little systemic anesthetic use. Any of the AE collected were considered as serious, although a significant difference in the onset of intraoperative delirium was found among groups (3 patients in group I vs 0 patients in group II. p=0.034). In general, scalp nerve blockade without supplemental systemic anesthetics could decrease the incidence of intraoperative neuropsychiatric adverse events and the length of the surgery [38].

Although scalp block is usually associated with decreased postoperative opioid consumption [39] and decreased opioid-related adverse events (post-operative nausea and vomiting - PONV- among others), some studies have shown no clinical significant advantage associated with its use. Gazoni et al studied 30 patients schedule to undergo craniotomy under standard general anesthesia. Based on the scalp block administration after the induction of GA, patients were randomized into two groups (receivers/ nonreceivers). Authors did not report any significant differences between groups with respect to postoperative opioid consumption, PONV, and hemodynamic variations [40].

Non-common adverse events have been reported while using local anesthesia including severe hypertension and coronary artery vasospasm [41, 42]. Additionally, airway management during an "awaked" anesthetic technique should be considered. Stereotactic frame might represent a challenge during the surgery, limiting patients' airway access [6]. Specific disease-related considerations, such as PD and obesity, should be evaluated with respect to airway management. Intraoperative larynx related neuromuscular dysfunction has been described in PD patients, increasing the potential risk of aspiration [43].

4.2. General Anesthesia

General anesthesia (GA) remains the preferred technique in certain patient population such as children, patients with non-controlled anxiety disorders, chronic pain, coughing, and severe movement disorders. Secured airway is the major advantage of GA, one of the major disadvantages being the interference with MERs and macrostimulation; with this respect, LA would be preferred to GA. However, some patients simply are not comfortable under LA due to several reasons (e.g. prolonged off-phase or without medication before surgery). Fluchere et al reported the outcomes of 213 PD patients that underwent DBS surgery between 2000 and 2009 with a variation of GA, with levels of sedation carefully titrated throughout surgical stages. All patients received a controlled general anesthesia using propofol and mechanical ventilation. MRI was used to identify the location of the leads, whereas stereotactic marks and trajectories were determined by the same neurosurgeon. At this time, propofol infusion was discontinued and sevoflurane was used for maintenance of anesthesia, allowing ideal sedation levels for MERs. Follow-up assessments were performed by the same neurologist one year post-surgery (in 188 patients), with a five years follow-up accomplished in only 65 patients. Authors concluded that this particular anesthesia technique did not affect short-term and long-term motor outcomes [44].

Essential neuromonitoring during DBS surgery will rely on the capability of some anesthetic drugs, such as propofol, to decrease tissue responses to stimulation or to allow intraoperative mental tasks. However, a case report published in 2006 by Deogaonkar et al described a PD patient developing midazolam and propofol-induced dyskinesia highlighting one of the undesirable effects of propofol [45].

Raz et al compared STN spiking activity in 16 PD patients alternating the exposure to propofol infusion. Once the electrodes were in place, traces of the STN were taken before and after the propofol infusion (50μg/kg/min). Low levels of sedation were accomplished within 11.9 ± 3.0 minutes, recorded either by Entropy (response and state entropy) or bispectral index (BIS), as well as capability of patients to respond to their names. STN activity is decreased in the presence of propofol infusion when comparing with baseline. Nevertheless, spiking activity returned to the baseline levels after 17 minutes from the time of propofol discontinuation [46].

Avoiding drugs that potentiate GABAergic transmission, such as propofol, may offer potential benefits during MERs [46, 47]. However, GA with propofol-remifentanil combination and successful identification of the subthalamic nucleus (STN) involving MERs and MRI techniques have been reported. This kind of anesthesia management requires an exceptional communication among anesthesiologists and the surgical team in order to achieve the expected goals through a close titration of anesthetic drugs [48].

4.3. Monitored anesthesia care

MAC is defined as a technique where local anesthesia is combined either with sedation (occasionally named as "conscious sedation") or with analgesia to obtain minimal changes in patients' consciousness, with response to verbal stimuli and spontaneous ventilation [49].

Electrophysiological evaluations during DBS surgery such as MERs and macrostimulation require an awake patient or the use of low levels of sedation. Dexmedetomidine is a well-known medication that has been used in anesthesia for more than 20 years with a distinctive effect at subcortical areas, producing ideal levels of sedation without respiratory impairments [1]. The ability to significantly decrease other anesthetic requirements, such as propofol and remifentanil, makes this α-2-adrenergic agonist the drug of choice for DBS surgery as a part of the MAC technique. Pharmacodynamic and pharmacokinetic properties of these drugs allow big changes in the level of sedation in a short period of time [50]. Usually, high level of sedation or even general anesthesia is required for fixation of pins and for the insertion of the generator (last step), lower levels being used during intraoperative assessment of stimulation [1].

Respiratory complications (e.g., desaturation and airway obstruction) are the most feared during MAC, due to their association with devastating irreversible consequences [1, 6].

5. Future of deep brain stimulation: anesthesia guidelines

New technologies developed during the past 70 years impacted DBS surgery and patient outcomes. Researchers and physicians are encouraged to design prospective studies on DBS in different clinical settings. New stem cells investigational therapies in neurocognitive dysfunction evaluate the quality of outcomes using DBS as a baseline tool [51].

Anesthesia protocol is centered on patient comorbidities such as neuromuscular impairment for PD or morbid obesity cases where hypoventilation and difficult airway are the main concerns. Guidelines for DBS anesthesia should be elaborated based on the feedback provided by experienced anesthesiologists. Anesthesia in functional neurosurgery should be correlated with surgical goals, providing adequate combinations of anesthetic drugs with minimal impact on neurological monitoring, and contributing to patient comfort and safety.

Author details

Juan Fiorda-Diaz[1*], Nicoleta Stoicea[1], Milind S. Deogaonkar[2] and Sergio D. Bergese[1,2]

*Address all correspondence to: Juan.Fiorda@osumc.edu

1 Department of Anesthesiology, The Ohio State University Wexner Medical Center, Columbus, Ohio, USA

2 Department of Neurosurgery, The Ohio State University Wexner Medical Center, Columbus, Ohio, USA

References

[1] Rozet, I., *Anesthesia for functional neurosurgery: the role of dexmedetomidine*. Curr Opin Anaesthesiol, 2008. 21(5): p. 537–43.

[2] Gionfriddo, M.R., et al., *Pathways of Translation: Deep Brain Stimulation*. Clinical and translational science, 2013. 6(6): p. 497–501.

[3] Vitek, J.L., *Mechanisms of deep brain stimulation: excitation or inhibition*. Movement disorders, 2002. 17(S3): p. S69–S72.

[4] Velasco, F., et al., *Metabolic Changes Induced by Electrical Stimulation of Prelemniscal Radiations for the Treatment of Parkinson Disease*. Stereotact Funct Neurosurg, 2015. 93(5): p. 333–41.

[5] Lozano, A.M. and N. Lipsman, *Probing and regulating dysfunctional circuits using deep brain stimulation*. Neuron, 2013. 77(3): p. 406–424.

[6] Chakrabarti, R., M. *Ghazanwy, and A. Tewari, Anesthetic challenges for deep brain stimulation: a systematic approach*. N Am J Med Sci, 2014. 6(8): p. 359–69.

[7] Grant, R., S.E. Gruenbaum, and J. Gerrard, *Anaesthesia for deep brain stimulation: a review*. Current Opinion in Anesthesiology, 2015. 28(5): p. 505–510.

[8] Venkatraghavan, L., et al., *Anesthesia for functional neurosurgery: review of complications*. Journal of neurosurgical anesthesiology, 2006. 18(1): p. 64–67.

[9] Beric, A., et al., *Complications of deep brain stimulation surgery*. Stereotact Funct Neurosurg, 2001. 77(1–4): p. 73–8.

[10] Sironi, V.A., *Origin and evolution of deep brain stimulation*. The development of deep brain stimulation for neurological and psychiatric disorders: clinical, societal and ethical issues, 2011: p. 4.

[11] Hariz, M.I., P. Blomstedt, and L. Zrinzo, *Deep brain stimulation between 1947 and 1987: the untold story*. Neurosurgical focus, 2010. 29(2): p. E1.

[12] Benabid, A.L., et al., Long-term suppression of tremor by chronic stimulation of the ventral intermediate thalamic nucleus. The Lancet, 1991. 337(8738): p. 403–406.

[13] Udupa, K. and R. Chen, *The mechanisms of action of deep brain stimulation and ideas for the future development*. Progress in neurobiology, 2015. 133: p. 27–49.

[14] Kobayashi, S. and A. Morita, *The History of Neuroscience and Neurosurgery in Japan*. 2015. (In Press):e867.

[15] Lozano, A.M., et al., *Subcallosal cingulate gyrus deep brain stimulation for treatment-resistant depression*. Biological psychiatry, 2008. 64(6): p. 461–467.

[16] Mirzadeh, Z., et al., *Validation of CT-MRI fusion for intraoperative assessment of stereotactic accuracy in DBS surgery*. Movement Disorders, 2014. 29(14): p. 1788–1795.

[17] Bronstein, J.M., et al., *Deep brain stimulation for Parkinson disease: an expert consensus and review of key issues*. Archives of neurology, 2011. 68(2): p. 165–165.

[18] Grant, R.A., et al., *Ethical considerations in deep brain stimulation for psychiatric illness*. Journal of Clinical Neuroscience, 2014. 21(1): p. 1–5.

[19] Pisapia, J.M., et al., *Ethical considerations in deep brain stimulation for the treatment of addiction and overeating associated with obesity*. AJOB Neuroscience, 2013. 4(2): p. 35–46.

[20] Nuttin, B., et al., *Consensus on guidelines for stereotactic neurosurgery for psychiatric disorders*. Journal of Neurology, Neurosurgery & Psychiatry, 2014. 85(9): p. 1003–1008.

[21] Benabid, A., et al., *Combined (thalamotomy and stimulation) stereotactic surgery of the VIM thalamic nucleus for bilateral Parkinson disease*. Stereotactic and functional neurosurgery, 1988. 50(1–6): p. 344–346.

[22] Deuschl, G., et al., *A randomized trial of deep-brain stimulation for Parkinson's disease*. New England Journal of Medicine, 2006. 355(9): p. 896–908.

[23] Montgomery, E.B., Jr., *Deep brain stimulation for hyperkinetic disorders*. Neurosurg Focus, 2004. 17(1): p. E1.

[24] Boccard, S.G., et al., *Long-term outcomes of deep brain stimulation for neuropathic pain*. Neurosurgery, 2013. 72(2): p. 221–30; discussion 231.

[25] Laxton, A.W., et al., *A phase I trial of deep brain stimulation of memory circuits in Alzheimer's disease*. Annals of neurology, 2010. 68(4): p. 521–534.

[26] Sankar, T., et al., *Deep brain stimulation influences brain structure in Alzheimer's disease*. Brain stimulation, 2015. 8(3): p. 645–654.

[27] Hescham, S., et al., *Deep brain stimulation of the forniceal area enhances memory functions in experimental dementia: the role of stimulation parameters*. Brain stimulation, 2013. 6(1): p. 72–77.

[28] Al–Harbi, K.S., *Treatment-resistant depression: therapeutic trends, challenges, and future directions*. Patient Prefer Adherence, 2012. 6: p. 369–388.

[29] Cleary, D.R., et al., *Deep brain stimulation for psychiatric disorders: where we are now*. Neurosurg Focus, 2015. 38(6): p. E2.

[30] Hamani, C., et al., *Deep brain stimulation for obsessive-compulsive disorder: systematic review and evidence-based guideline sponsored by the American Society for Stereotactic and Functional Neurosurgery and the Congress of Neurological Surgeons (CNS) and endorsed by the CNS and American Association of Neurological Surgeons*. Neurosurgery, 2014. 75(4): p. 327–33; quiz 333.

[31] Fryar, C.D., M.D. Carroll, and C.L. Ogden, *Prevalence of overweight, obesity, and extreme obesity among adults: United States, trends 1960–1962 through 2009–2010*. Hyattsville, MD: National Center for Health Statistics, 2012.

[32] Hamani, C., et al., *Memory enhancement induced by hypothalamic/fornix deep brain stimulation*. Annals of neurology, 2008. 63(1): p. 119–123.

[33] Taghva, A., J.D. Corrigan, and A.R. Rezai, *Obesity and brain addiction circuitry: implications for deep brain stimulation*. Neurosurgery, 2012. 71(2): p. 224–38.

[34] Abosch, A., et al., *An international survey of deep brain stimulation procedural steps.* Stereotactic and functional neurosurgery, 2012. 91(1): p. 1–11.

[35] Warnke, P.C., *Deep brain stimulation surgery under general anaesthesia with microelectrode recording: the best of both worlds or a little bit of everything?* Journal of Neurology, Neurosurgery & Psychiatry, 2014. 85(10): p. 1063–1063.

[36] Scharpf, D.T., et al., *Practical considerations and nuances in anesthesia for patients undergoing deep brain stimulation implantation surgery.* Korean J Anesthesiol, 2015. 68(4): p. 332–9.

[37] Hansen, E., et al., *Awake craniotomies without any sedation: the awake-awake-awake technique.* Acta neurochirurgica, 2013. 155(8): p. 1417–1424.

[38] Lange, M., et al., *Anesthesiologic regimen and intraoperative delirium in deep brain stimulation surgery for Parkinson's disease.* J Neurol Sci, 2015. 355(1–2): p. 168–73.

[39] Hwang, J.-Y., et al., *Effect of scalp blocks with levobupivacaine on recovery profiles after craniotomy for aneurysm clipping: a randomized, double-blind, and controlled study.* World neurosurgery, 2013.

[40] Gazoni, F.M., N. Pouratian, and E.C. Nemergut, *Effect of ropivacaine skull block on perioperative outcomes in patients with supratentorial brain tumors and comparison with remifentanil: a pilot study.* 2008.

[41] Yamada, K., et al., *Stereotactic surgery for subthalamic nucleus stimulation under general anesthesia: a retrospective evaluation of Japanese patients with Parkinson's disease.* Parkinsonism & related disorders, 2007. 13(2): p. 101–107.

[42] Glossop, A. and P. Dobbs, *Coronary artery vasospasm during awake deep brain stimulation surgery.* British journal of anaesthesia, 2008. 101(2): p. 222–224.

[43] Khatib, R., et al., *Perioperative events during deep brain stimulation: the experience at Cleveland clinic.* Journal of neurosurgical anesthesiology, 2008. 20(1): p. 36–40.

[44] Fluchere, F., et al., *Controlled general anaesthesia for subthalamic nucleus stimulation in Parkinson's disease.* Journal of Neurology, Neurosurgery & Psychiatry, 2013: p. jnnp-2013–305323.

[45] Deogaonkar, A., et al., *Propofol-induced dyskinesias controlled with dexmedetomidine during deep brain stimulation surgery.* The Journal of the American Society of Anesthesiologists, 2006. 104(6): p. 1337–1339.

[46] Raz, A., et al., *Propofol decreases neuronal population spiking activity in the subthalamic nucleus of Parkinsonian patients.* Anesthesia & Analgesia, 2010. 111(5): p. 1285–1289.

[47] Hippard, H.K., et al., *Preservation of microelectrode recordings with non–GABAergic drugs during deep brain stimulator placement in children: Technical note.* Journal of Neurosurgery: Pediatrics, 2014. 14(3): p. 279–286.

[48] Hertel, F., et al., *Implantation of electrodes for deep brain stimulation of the subthalamic nucleus in advanced Parkinson's disease with the aid of intraoperative microrecording under general anesthesia*. Neurosurgery, 2006. 59(5): p. E1138; discussion E1138.

[49] Ghisi, D., et al., *Monitored anesthesia care*. Minerva Anestesiol, 2005. 71(9): p. 533–8.

[50] Jani, J.M., C.O. Oluigbo, and S.K. Reddy, *Anesthesia for deep brain stimulation in traumatic brain injury-induced hemidystonia*. Clinical case reports, 2015. 3(6): p. 492–495.

[51] Barker, R.A. and I. de Beaufort, *Scientific and ethical issues related to stem cell research and interventions in neurodegenerative disorders of the brain*. Progress in neurobiology, 2013. 110: p. 63–73.

Chapter 2

Deep Brain Stimulation: The Perspective of Brain Connectivity

Hae Yu Kim

Additional information is available at the end of the chapter

http://dx.doi.org/10.5772/62829

Abstract

Deep brain stimulation (DBS) has been demonstrated as a treatment option to alleviate patient symptoms in movement disorders, such as Parkinson's disease (PD) and dystonia, and has emerged as an alternative treatment for medically intractable epilepsy. However, complete understanding of the mechanism of DBS remains elusive despite recent human and nonhuman studies that have provided mechanistic clues. The precise mechanisms of action for DBS remain unclear. This review provides an up-to-date overview of the detailed procedures of DBS and reviews the actions of DBS on brain networks. Studies regarding the structural and functional connectivity of the brain are also reviewed.

Keywords: Deep brain stimulation, Mechanism, Structural brain connectivity, Functional brain connectivity, brain network

1. Introduction

In previous decades, the function of deep brain stimulation (DBS) has been demonstrated as the activation or inhibition of specific brain regions, which are the targets of DBS [1, 2]. It has been suggested that the mechanism of DBS must be an inhibition of an area of a pathological network in the brain because the clinical results for DBS are similar or better than classical ablation therapy. However, we soon had to admit that it is not an activation/inhibition problem of a specific brain region, but rather the neuromodulation of brain networks [3–5]. The concepts of brain network neuromodulation were based on the idea that DBS represents not only remarkable therapeutic benefits for patients but also an amazingly powerful research tool to interrogate brain networks. Specifically, the underlying brain function may be demonstrated if DBS is used in conjunction with noninvasive neuroimaging methods, such as magnetoencephalography (MEG), electroencephalography (EEG), and functional imaging modalities.

In previous decades, studies regarding the structural and functional brain networks have nourished us in terms of how DBS works. Nevertheless, the knowledge regarding the structural networks of the brain was cruel and so were the functional networks. The structural networks of the brain have been investigated with various modalities [3, 5–8]. Furthermore, studies have been extended toward functional brain connectivity via investigations with models based on MEG and EEG [9, 10]. Recently, an emerging trial has been attempted to connect structural and functional brain connectivity and understand the genuine brain networks [4, 11].

This review provides us an up-to-date overview of the detailed procedures of DBS and monitoring during surgery, as well as reviews the actions of DBS on brain networks based on human and nonhuman studies. Furthermore, studies regarding the structural and functional connectivity of the brain are also reviewed.

2. Deep brain stimulation

2.1. Historical review

DBS is a surgical option that has not arisen de novo. It has resulted from a gradual evolution. The first trial reported to modulate brain function via electrical brain stimulation was in 1870 [12]. Electrical stimulation of the motor cortex in a dog provoked limb movement. Sir Victor Horsley, the father of functional neurosurgery, first performed intraoperative brain stimulation in 1884 [13]. He demonstrated conjugational eyeball movement via electrical stimulation of the corpora quadrigemina within an occipital encephalocele. Modern style stereotactic electrical stimulation in humans was conducted by Spiegel et al. [14] in 1947, which was approximately 30 years after the invention of the first animal stereotactic apparatus in 1908 by Horsley and Clark [15]. The first human case exhibited Huntington's disease. The authors used brain stimulation to identify the correct position of the lesion within the brain. Stereotactic brain stimulation subsequently continued to be used in nearly every stereotactic surgery because its purpose was to ensure the position of the lesioning electrode.

As stereotactic brain surgery progressed, it was recognized that brain stimulation within the target may have a mimicking effect with the target lesioning. Hassler et al. [16] reported that the stimulation of the ventral lateral (subsequently referred to as the ventral intermediate nucleus of thalamus (VIM)) nucleus of the thalamus during stereotactic localization may terminate the tremor. Furthermore, Alberts et al. [17] reported that dystonic symptoms improved following stimulation during stereotactic surgery. Delgado et al. [18] introduced electrode implantation in human brains as a technique for chronic recording and brain stimulation, and Heath [19] initiated depth electrode studies for psychotic patients in the 1950s.

Mortimer and Shealy became involved in an implantable stimulator in Medtronics in 1965, and the base of the DBS system was founded [20]. Shealy et al. [21] implanted the first dorsal column stimulator in 1967, and, thereafter, the neuromodulation for pain was actively performed. The early stimulators at this time comprised two parts, including an implantable passive receiver and a battery-controlled external device. The two parts were coupled by radiofrequency and transmitted both control and power. In 1981, Medtronic released a completely implanted stimulator. In the mid-1970s, Cooper et al. [22, 23] introduced cerebellar cortical stimulation for the treatment of epilepsy and cerebral palsy.

In 1973, Hosobuchi et al. [24] stereotactically implanted a DBS electrode in the somatosensory thalamus to treat denervation pain. It had previously been recognized that stimulation during surgery could mimic the effects of lesioning from the early era of stereotactic surgery; however, the mechanism was not fully understood [25]. The target of DBS to treat movement disorders naturally originated from the target of ablation surgery. Brice and McLellan [26] first reported DBS for movement disorder in 1980. The patient was suffering intentional tremor with no pain because of multiple sclerosis. They implanted the electrode in the thalamus to control the tremor. In 1986, Siegfried [27] demonstrated an improvement of dyskinesia in a patient with pain caused by Dejerin-Roussy syndrome, which had undergone DBS implantation to treat the pain. Benabid et al. [1] introduced the use of chronic VIM stimulation for the treatment of Parkinsonian tremor. Finally, high-frequency stimulation was used at any targets that were used for lesioning in the 1980s.

Hesitation remained to implement DBS for Parkinson's disease (PD) at this time because physicians preferred medical management with L-dopa and related drugs. However, the surgical management of PD was reborn following the reintroduction of pallidotomy in 1992 [28]. DBS was also reintroduced with the same target in 1994, and several neurosurgeons subsequently popularized it [29–31]. Benabid has attempted to elucidate the mechanisms of DBS for movement disorders and to make it widely accepted. He also reported bilateral subthalamic nucleus (STN) stimulation for PD [32]. Forel's field and zona inserta have been suggested as novel targets, in addition to the STN and globus pallidus internus (GPi). To date, DBS has returned toward the era of brain lesioning for psychological conditions and epilepsy. Moreover, it has not only accepted all old targets with the fundamentals obtained through human and nonhuman investigations but has also expanded new targets from vigorous investigation.

2.2. Surgical indication

DBS is most commonly used to alleviate the motor symptoms of PD despite initial implementation to treat intractable pain. It may be used for the treatment of dystonia and essential tremor. Furthermore, it is in limited use or under investigation to treat various neurological and psychological conditions, including epilepsy, obsessive-compulsive disorder (OCD), and major depression. DBS has opened new horizons for the surgical treatment of various neurological and psychiatric conditions [33]. The spark to extend the clinical indications has expanded to investigational research on neurological, psychological, cognitive, and behavioral conditions. **Table 1** comprises a summary of the surgical indications for DBS according to the symptoms that require treatment.

Indications	Medical conditions
Parkinsonism (tremor, bradykinesia, and rigidity)	Idiopathic Parkinson's disease
Tremors	Parkinson's disease (only tremor dominant), Essential tremor, *Rubral tremor, posttraumatic tremor*
Dystonic movement	Primary dystonia, *Secondary dystonia*
Dyskinesia	Parkinson's disease (Dopamine-induced dyskinesia), Tardive dyskinesia
Chorea	*Huntington's chorea*
Seizures	Intractable epilepsy as a result of many cause
Mood	Major depression
Obsession	Obsessive compulsive disorder
Tics	Tourette's syndrome
Pain	Chronic pain, *Cluster headache*
Obesity	*Eating disorder*
Anorexia nervosa	*Eating disorder*
Cognitive failure	*Alzheimer's disease, Severe traumatic brain injury*
Addiction	*Psychological cause*
Tinnitus	*Uncontrollable otological problem*

Limited use or investigational state in italics.

Table 1. Summary of symptoms for treatment via DBS.

2.3. Optimal targets of DBS

Successful surgical results of DBS definitely originated from the optimal target according to the specific symptoms or disease entities. For example, the classical target for tremor has been the VIM of the thalamus since the era of stereotactic brain lesioning. However, Parkinsonian tremor has also been controlled with other Parkinsonian symptoms via STN stimulation. Moreover, many surgeons have often targeted the GPi to treat patients with predominately dopamine-induced dyskinesia with minimal tremor [34]. Some authors recommend the GPi better than the STN for patients with postural instability and gait disturbance as indicated by a meta-analysis [35]. Randomized controlled studies have not concluded which target is better for PD patients [36–38]. Moreover, there is no general consensus regarding the best target, the STN or GPi. Consequently, the choice of best target for an individual patient may depend on the conditions the patient has suffered.

As DBS widened its clinical indications, new targets have continuously emerged. Ethical problems have been associated with new targets; however, vigorous investigation regarding the new targets has been performed through nonhuman experiments to prove its efficacy and safety. **Table 2** shows the targets published to date regarding whether they are established or investigational.

Indications	Targets
Parkinsonism (tremor, bradykinesia, and rigidity)	STN, GPi, and PPN
Tremors	VIM
Dystonic movement	GPi
Dyskinesia	GPi
Chorea	*GPi*
Seizures	ANT, DMT, *Hippocampus, Cerebellum*
Mood	*GPi (anteromedial), NA, Anterior capsule, Medial thalamic structure, Prefrontal cortex, Cingulum, Dorsolateral prefrontal cortex, Inferior thalamic peduncle, Prefrontal cortex, Ventral striatum, Zona inserta (medial part)*
Obsession	*NA, Anterior capsule, Bed nucleus of stria terminalis, interior thalamic peduncle, STN (limbic part), ventral striatum*
Tics	*GPi (posteroventral), STN, NA, Anteromeidal pallidus internus, CMpf, Voi, Ventral striatum*
Pain	Vpm/Vpl, Motor cortex, *PAG/PVG, posteromedial hypothalamus*
Obesity	*Lateral hypothalamus*
Anorexia nervosa	*Subgenual cingulum*
Cognitive failure	*Nucleus basalis of Meynert, fornix, entorhinal area, medial thalamus*
Addiction	*NA*
Tinnitus	*VIM*

Limited use or investigational state in italics. ANT, anterior nucleus of thalamus; CMpf, centeromedin parafasciculus of thalamus; DMT, dorsomedial nucleus of thalamus; NA, nucleus accumbens; PAG/PVG, periaqueductal gray/periventricular gray; STN, subthalamic nucleus; GPi, globus pallidus internus; PPN, pedunculopontine nucleus; VIM, ventral intermediate nucleus of thalamus; Vpm/Vpl, ventral posteromedian/ventral posterolateral thalamus.

Table 2. DBS targets previously published.

2.4. Surgical procedures of DBS

Advanced surgical skills are not necessary to perform DBS. However, the flow of surgical procedures should be well acquainted. The author would like to divide the flow of surgical procedures into five steps because there are common steps of all DBS procedures and different steps depending on the specific target of DBS. Moreover, the author would like to introduce what the author is doing and include several tips that other authors have recommended in the literature.

2.4.1. Preoperative step

The clinical decision regarding whether DBS may be helpful for a specific patient is critical. Prior to this decision, an exact diagnosis is necessary using a multidisciplinary approach. Most movement disorders are clinically diagnosed, which implies a small portion of uncertainty. Nevertheless, an exact diagnosis may inform the surgeons, as well as the patients and their families regarding the expected results of DBS. The author highly recommends organizing a team that comprises a neurologist, neuropsychiatrist, neuropsychologist, anesthesiologist, and special nurse (may vary from institute to institute) in your institute to discuss and confirm the diagnosis and clinical indications. In the case of PD, an L-dopa challenge test is necessary to confirm DBS. The PD patient may need to be hospitalized for this test for several days.

Once the decision is made, the patient undergoes the surgical procedures. Patients considered for DBS must be hospitalized for several days. In the case of PD, antiparkinsonian medication should be terminated for 4–12 h according to the duration of the on-time prior to the start of surgery. Too early cessation of antiparkinsonian medication will cause substantial discomfort. On the day of surgery, the stereotactic frame was applied following a local anesthesia injection at four pinning sites. The author uses a Leksell G stereotactic frame. Cosman-Roberts-Wells (CRW) or other stereotactic frames may also be used. The stereotactic frame should be applied parallel to the line from the nose ring to the tragus. The author recommends that the accuracy of the stereotactic frame should be checked regularly as recommended by the manufacturer. Frameless DBS is currently performed in some institutes with reported results and accuracy [39–41]. These authors have indicated that the accuracy is the same as previous frame-based DBS, and the choice should be based on surgeon preference.

The patient is subsequently transferred to the MRI room. The patient's head with frame is fixed to the adaptor of a 1.5 T MRI. The MRI scan is performed, including 1 mm T1-weighted axial images with gadolinium enhancement (recommend double-dosed enhancement) and 2 mm T2-weighted axial images. If the condition is allowed, 2 mm T2-weighted coronal images may be obtained (may be optionally fused with T2 axial images, described later in the Targeting step). In some institutes, MRI is performed on the day prior to surgery, and computed tomography (CT) is conducted after frame application on the day of surgery. MRI is subsequently performed on the previous day and is fused before targeting [42]. Some authors recommend contrasted CT because of the vessel visualization issue [43, 44]. This approach is completely based on surgeon preference. The patient is transferred to the operating room to prepare for the surgical step.

2.4.2. Targeting step

All MRI images are transferred to a Leksell Surgiplan workstation (Elekta, Sweden). The author also uses FrameLink (Medtronics, Minneapolis, USA) and believes that there is no

http://dx.doi.org/10.5772/62829

specific difference that affects the surgical results. There may be other planning stations depending on the institutes. First, the anterior commissure (AC) and posterior commissure (PC), which are the anterior and posterior extremes, respectively, of the third ventricle, should be identified in T1 axial and sagittal images. The AC–PC line-based target coordinates are defined in the T2-weighted images, depending on the target at the time of surgery decision. At this time, T2-weighted axial and coronal images are fused if these are available. The author feels that this work may minimize the distortion error of the MRI images even though the distortion error of a 1.5 T MRI image is within the acceptable boundary [45]. The targets, such as the STN and GPi, may be easily visualized on T-2 weighted MRI images (**Figure 1**). However, the author first defines the target using formulated coordinates and subsequently adjusts it in the case of the STN and GPi. After the target is defined, trajectory from the cortical entry point will be defined. The recommended entry point is the middle frontal gyrus, and the visualized vessels should be avoided. Furthermore, the trajectory through the ventricle should be avoided. At this point, adjustment of the target may be necessary because a different trajectory may modify the optimal penetration of the target. Maximal options may be used for the stimulation sites, and optimal results may be expected when the electrode covers the maximal area of the target. Some authors have first defined the trajectory, followed by the target. The author thinks that the order between the trajectory and target does not matter because some adjustment should be followed according to the vessel positions and the best penetration of the target. **Table 3** shows the common target coordinates of DBS.

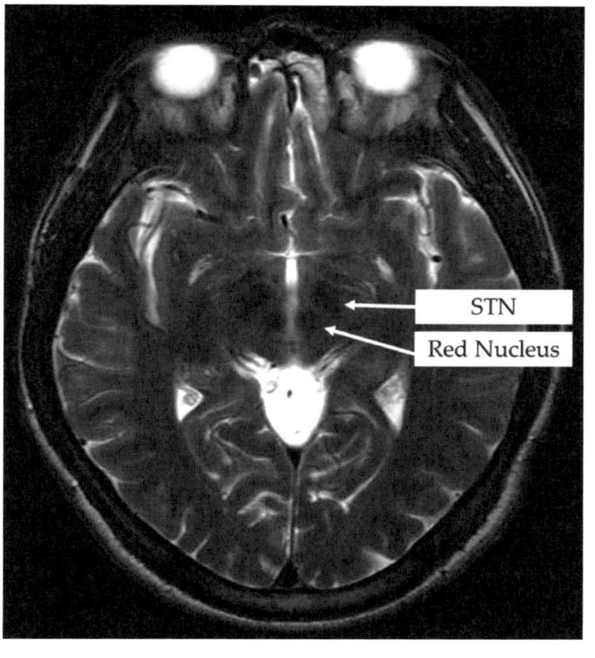

Figure 1. T2-weighted axial MR image indicates red nucleus and subthalamic nucleus.

	STN	GPi	VIM	Vpm/Vpl	NA
AC–PC line	50%	50%	28.5% anterior	33.4% anterior	100% anterior
Vertical	2–4 mm inferior	4 mm inferior	0	0	1–3 mm inferior
Lateral	11–13 mm	20–22 mm	12–15 mm	11–14 mm	6–9 mm
Axial	1–3 mm posterior	1–2 mm anterior	0	0	7–9 mm anterior

NA, nucleus accumbens; STN, subthalamic nucleus; GPi, globus pallidus internus; VIM, ventral intermediate nucleus of thalamus; Vpm/Vpl, ventral posteromedian/ventral posterolateral thalamus.

Table 3. Decisions regarding common targets of DBS.

2.4.3. Operative step

The patient is positioned supine, and a stereotactic frame is fixed to a special headrest. The patient's head and upper body may be elevated, and the knees are slightly flexed on the pillows. This sitting-like position is for the patient's comfort and is helpful to minimize the flowing out of cerebrospinal fluid (CSF) through the burr holes during surgery. Prior to draping, special monitoring may be needed, for example, EEG for an epilepsy case and EMG for a movement disorder case. Absolute separation of the sterile area from the nonsterile area is critical. The author uses a transverse metal bar and a large transparent drape that exposes only the upper area of both sidebars of the stereotactic frame. A double-check of the target coordinates by two neurosurgeons are highly recommended. A neurologist or special nurse should be present during surgery by the patient's side, in the opposite area from the surgical field. The intracranial electrode implantation is performed under local anesthesia. A local anesthetic injection is administered around the skin incision marks after the trajectory is set with the correct target coordinates. The author prefers curvilinear skin incisions to avoid skin erosion complications [46]. A burr hole is made with a pneumatic perforator, and bleeding was completely controlled. An incision on the dura mater is subsequently performed and completely coagulated. A corticotomy follows with specific attention on avoiding the vessels and sulcus. At this point, when the dura mater is opened, normal blood pressure and normal intracranial pressure should be confirmed. If the patient is not calm, brain-penetrating procedures may be extremely harmful. Once the outer cannula is inserted, the burr hole should be sealed to avoid CSF outflow [47]. Prior to the introduction of the microelectrode recording (MER) electrode, the patient should be neurologically examined by a neurologist or a special nurse.

The MER electrode is descended 10 mm above the target. The MER was checked every 1 mm and should be 0.5 mm or less than 5 mm above the target. In the case of PD, a typical MER finding of the STN may be identified, and the MER is typically descended to the substantia nigra pars reticulate (SNr). In the case of dystonia, a typical GPi firing may be identified, and the descent of the MER continued to the optic tract. The length of the target that the MER electrode penetrates is checked, and the selection of the current trajectory and the depth of intracranial electrode contact are subsequently decided. The author prefers a single track MER rather than a multichannel (e.g., Ben gun) MER system and believes that there is no difference in the results [48]. A test-stimulation is subsequently conducted via the MER electrode. The author checked the clinical effect during the stimulation and the side effects related to the stimulation. In the case of epilepsy, EEG changes, i.e., driving response or recruiting rhythm, may be identified during low frequency stimulation of the thalamus during test-stimulation [49, 50]. If the test-stimulation is satisfactory, a permanent electrode is introduced toward the previously decided depth under fluoroscopy. The final trajectory and position of the electrode should be decided by three aspects; first, the exact image-guided target; second, the proper MER finding; and third, an adequate physiological response to the test-stimulation. After the electrode is introduced, test-stimulation via the permanent electrode is performed to confirm the correct position. If it is satisfactory, the electrode is fixed with a special fixing system of the DBS system with attention paid to the depth of electrode under fluoroscopy. The same procedure would be performed on the other side.

The patient is transferred to the CT room without removing the stereotactic frame. A CT scan is performed at 1 mm without enhancement to confirm the position of the electrode and intracranial hemorrhage. The CT images are transferred to the same workstation used for the target planning. After the exact electrode position is confirmed with an image fusion technique, the patient's frame is removed. Implantable pulse generators (IPG) were subsequently inserted into the bilateral subclavian area under general anesthesia. There are several options to perform DBS, i.e., bilateral simultaneous intracranial electrode insertion and IPG insertion on the same day, unilateral intracranial electrode insertion and same side IPG insertion on the same day, bilateral intracranial electrode insertion on one day and subsequent IPG insertion on another day, and unilateral intracranial electrode insertion on one day and subsequent IPG insertion on another day. These options are all successful and may be different depending on the surgeon's preference, patient's condition, and other various health system logistics [42, 51–56].

2.4.4. Postoperative step

The patient is transferred to the recovery room following the insertion of the IPG ends. Following recovery from anesthesia, the patient is transferred to the neurological ward. Surgery-related issues are considered during hospitalization. First, surgical infection related to hardware may be an issue. Prophylactic antibiotics are initiated from the preoperative stage to postoperative 2–3 days. The surgical wound should be closely followed thorough the wound healing course. The author recommends that stitches are removed 9–10 days after surgery. Hospitalization is not required for this entire period. The inpatient period depends on the condition of the patient. Second, a microlesional effect of DBS (transient and irregular symptomatic improvement after DBS) may be an issue. Most patients who underwent DBS experience an improvement of preoperative symptoms without stimulation. The period of microlesional effect varies by patient; however, it typically lasts from days to weeks. Medications, especially anti-parkinsonian medications, should be decreased according to the patient's symptom improvement during this period. Third, the timing of stimulation may be an issue. The author recommends that the stimulation is initiated 4–6 weeks after surgery. The reasons are that stable effects of stimulation cannot be expected without full recovery of the patient's condition and microlesional effects disturb the tuning of the stimulation parameters. Fourth, delirium or other psychological symptoms in limited patients, such as old aged PD, may be an issue [57]. These symptoms typically last 3–7 days after surgery and may result in an extension of the hospital period. The symptoms are easily controlled with tranquilizers; however, a special psychological consultation may be needed.

2.4.5. Outpatient follow-up step

During the outpatient follow-up step, the most important issue is the initiation of stimulation. As the author previously mentioned, stimulation will be initiated 4–6 weeks after surgery. The author recommends that the patient may require hospitalization for 1–2 days unless the outpatient department provides sufficient room to check the patient's walking and whole movements with trial-and-error based stimulation and sufficient time to wait for patient's symptom changes with stimulation. The author prefers a shorter follow-up (1–2 weeks) during the early simulation period for fine-tuning of the stimulation with an adjustment of medication. Regular follow-up may subsequently be continued with the neurologist or the neurosurgeon every 6–8 weeks. Neuropsychological tests and other special studies, such as EEG and video movement evaluation, may be conducted every 1–2 years. The institute where DBS is performed should construct a system (via telephone or in person) for the patients to contact any time if they have concerns related to DBS.

2.5. Clinical results

Essential tremor is the most common movement disorder. VIM DBS is the most commonly used target for this condition. Long-term follow-up studies have demonstrated a 40–80% reduction in the tremor severity and corresponding improvement in the quality of life [58–65]. **Table 4** shows the results of 1 year and longer follow-up studies on VIM DBS for essential tremor [63, 65–68]. Approximately 10% of patients do not have adequate tremor control with VIM DBS. Furthermore, approximately 15% of patients initially improve, but subsequently lose efficacy within one year after surgery [69].

PD is the most well-published disease entity. All publications have used the medically validated unified Parkinson's disease rating scale (UPDRS), which comprises four components: Part I assesses changes in mentation and cognition (including behavior and mood); Part II assesses changes in daily living activities; Part III assesses motor symptoms; and Part IV assesses therapeutic complications [70]. Hoehn and Yahr [71] have also been used to assess the disease stage, as well as a PD questionnaire (the 39-item PD questionnaire, PDQ-39) to determine the quality of life [72]. The mainstay of PD management is medical therapy in the early stage and surgical therapy in the later stage of the disease. The goal of the therapy is to increase the dopamine level in the brain and/or prolong the effect of dopamine [73]. DBS and medical therapy have been compared in large controlled trials as showed in **Table 5** [74–76]. Most studies have reported that DBS is superior to medical therapy in improvements; however, DBS has more serious adverse events. The long-term results of DBS have also been reported [77–79]. **Table 6** shows the long-term results of STN DBS.

No. of patients	Follow-up	Tremor improvement	Publication year	Authors
37 (28 bilateral, 9 unilateral)	1 year	General 55%; head (bilateral only) 85%; arm 80%; leg 75%; ADL 80%; voice none	1999	Limousin et al.
27 (14 bilateral, 13 unilateral)	1 year	Unilateral: arm 82%; head 38%; voice none Bilateral: head 95%; voice 83%	2000	Obwegeser et al.
25	40.2 months	Overall tremor 50% at last follow-up	2001	Koller et al.
19	6–7 years	Upper extremity tremor reduction: 100% of patients at 2 years, 84% of patients at 6–7 years	2003	Rehnerone et al.
19 (12 bilateral, 7 unilateral)	6.5 years	General 41%; arm 50%; head (bilateral only) 85%; voice none	2003	Sydow et al.

Table 4. One year or more follow-up studies regarding VIM DBS for essential tremor.

No. of patients	Follow-up	Improvement	Adverse events	Publication year	Authors
124 STN DBS 127 Medical	2 years	DBS>Medical	54.8% DBS, 44.1% Medical of serious adverse events	2013	Schuepbach et al.
174 STN DBS 183 Medical	1 year	DBS>Medical	20 patients DBS, 13 patients Medical of serious adverse events	2010	Williams et al.
78 STN DBS 78 Medical	6 months	DBS>Medical	13% DBS, 4% Medical($p < 0.04$) of serious adverse events	2006	Deuschl et al.

Table 5. Comparison of DBS and medical therapy.

No. of patients	Follow-up	Motor improvement	L-dopa equivalent dose reduction	Publication year	Authors
14	9 years	UPDRS motor score: 42% ADL: no improvement Motor complication: 59%	39%	2011	Zibetti et al.
18	10 years	UPDRS motor score: better than baseline ($p = 0.007$)	significant	2011	Castrioto et al.
20	8 years	UPDRS motor score: better than baseline ($p < 0.001$)	60.3%	2010	Fasano et al.

Table 6. Long-term results of subthalamic nucleus DBS.

DBS for dystonia is also well published. The severity of dystonia is quantified by several rating scales, including the Burk–Fahn–Marsden dystonia rating scale (BFMDRS) for generalized dystonia, and the Toronto–Western Spasmodic Torticollis Rating Scale (TWSTRS) for cervical and craniocervical dystonia [80, 81]. Bilateral GPi DBS for generalized primary dystonia results in a 60–80% improvement in the BFMDRS in open-label studies and 40–50% improvement in prospective, double-blind, randomized trials with 6–12 months of follow-up [82–87]. Tardive dystonia, which represents secondary dystonia, has a favourable outcome with DBS in several small, open-label studies that indicate a 50–70% improvement [88, 89]. Primary cervical and craniocervical dystonias have fair results following DBS, with a 40 > 70% improvement in the TWSTRS [90–93].

2.6. Complications

2.6.1. Surgical procedure-related complications

The surgical procedure-related complications are more or less similar regardless of the diseases and targets of DBS. In general, the most devastating complication is intracerebral hemorrhage (ICH). The overall incidence of ICH during DBS, regardless of the amount of ICH, has been reported as 1–9% [94–99]. The condition of patients with ICH during surgery depends on the location and the amount of ICH. The author believes that symptomatic ICH accounts for less than 1% of all procedures, and the occurrence of permanent deficits is lower [100]. The author recommends that several variables should be completely considered; first, a careful evaluation of blood coagulation; second, the avoidance of visualized vessels during trajectory planning; third, blood pressure control during surgery; and four, the maintenance of patient calmness during surgery. There is no general consensus regarding whether the MER is related to ICH [101, 102]. Cerebral infarction occurs; however, it is extremely rare [103–106]. Other complications associated with permanent neurological deficits are postoperative delirium, seizures, and other complications in the patient's general state. These surgical procedure-related complications have not been correlated with the duration of surgery or the electrode passing number [96, 107–110].

2.6.2. *Hardware-related complications*

There are many reports regarding hardware related complications, and the incidence is quite high, i.e., 2.7–50% [86, 94, 95, 98, 99, 111–121]. Most complications are infections, and their occurrence rate is 1.1–15% of published cases. The infections are predominantly superficial, and only approximately 1% are severe. They typically occur within 3 months after surgery, and IPG sites are more common [97, 98, 108, 111, 114, 115]. Other hardware-related problems include erosions of skin, lead fracture, IPG malfunction, and premature IPG drain-out [97, 99, 108, 113, 122, 123]. These problems cause additional procedures or surgeries; however, they may be managed without permanent deficits. Minor hardware-related problems include discomfort around the extension lead and thickening of scars. Although it is extremely rare, head trauma may occur in patients with the DBS system. This issue has been reported, and there was no stimulation failure problem if the electrode location was maintained [124, 125].

2.6.3. *Stimulation-related complications*

Stimulation-related complications are common; however, permanent neurological problems induced by these complications are rare. Complications often occur if the electrode placement is suboptimum. The current through the electrode spreads to the neural tissue around the target if the electrode location is not separate from the eloquent tissue, and the stimulation provokes wanted neurological symptoms that vary according to the anatomical location [118, 120, 126, 127]. Common complications include dysarthria, dysphonia, paresthesia, motor contraction, eyeball deviation, visual flushes, nausea, dizziness, eyelid opening apraxia, sweating, and dyskinesia. The major advantage of DBS is the changeability of the stimulation parameters and contacts. Most stimulation-related problems are managed with an adjustment of stimulation. Some patients initially have no problem and subsequently develop stimulation-related complications as the stimulation parameters are progressively increased. This occurs in the optimal placement of the electrode; thus, the stimulation, drugs or both should be adjusted [75, 127, 128].

Alterations in higher brain functions have been reported in PD patients. Most patients who have cognitive or behavioral deterioration after surgery had similar symptoms prior to surgery [129]. Common symptoms include transient hypomania, acute sadness, impulsive aggressive behavior, hilarity, or mania, and these symptoms occur as a result of both drugs and STN DBS [75, 128, 130–133]. Suicide is an emerging concern in PD patients who underwent STN DBS [94, 129, 134]. However, depression and suicide are multifactorial, related to treatment change or related to social issues and are not specifically related to the procedure [135]. Mood changes after STN DBS may represent abnormal behaviors caused by abrupt changes in limbic STN activity [131].

3. Mechanism of DBS

To date, it is clear that DBS represents functionally reversible lesioning [136]. DBS has different clinical effect times according to the indications and targets [137]. For example, VIM DBS for essential tremor resulted in the disappearance of tremor within seconds [138]. STN DBS exhibited an improvement of tremor within seconds, an improvement of bradykinesia and rigidity within minutes to hours, and an improvement of axial symptoms within hours to days [139, 140]. Similar phenomena in which the clinical effect time varies were demonstrated when we turned on/off the stimulation and when we stimulated other targets for psychological problems and intractable epilepsy [140–145]. These different responses to DBS suggest that its mechanisms are complicated, i.e., immediate neuromodulation and synaptic plasticity and anatomical remodeling [137, 140].

3.1. Acute responses: immediate neuromodulation

Stimulation through the DBS electrode inserted into the target inhibits neurons near the electrode. This finding was classically demonstrated clinically and was also supported by the determination that neurochemical inhibition improved Parkinsonian signs in animal models [146, 147]. The inhibitory effect of DBS was explained via in vitro studies. High-frequency stimulation induced a depolarization block, i.e., a sustained depolarization of neuronal membranes, inactivation of sodium channels, and increase of potassium currents [148, 149]. Furthermore, DBS activates inhibitory presynaptic terminals on the afferents to the cell body. The inhibitory action occurs through the release of the inhibitory neurotransmitter gamma-aminobutyric acid (GABA) [150].

Axons and dendrites around the electrode are predominantly affected rather than the soma because of the substantially high threshold of the soma [151]. Consequently, neurons whose dendrites or axons are close to the electrode may be more readily activated [152]. The action potentials of the affected neurons propagate away from or toward the soma. Clinical physicians may identify the effects of DBS when they change the stimulation parameters, for example, by adjusting the number and configuration of the anode or cathode electrode contacts and the voltage or current of the stimulation. Furthermore, evidence suggests that DBS induces action potentials in the passing afferent fibers around the target [153, 154].

3.2. Chronic responses: plasticity and remodeling

DBS effects that emerge over a long period of time (days to months) may suggest that it changes neural networks. There is a report that STN stimulation in the rat brain induced various forms of synaptic plasticity in the STN neuronal subpopulation [155]. In dopamine-depleted rats, short-term depression and long-term depression were induced by high-frequency stimulation, and the effects of stimulation were abolished with the administration of dopamine agonist

[156]. This phenomenon suggested that stimulation-induced synaptic changes were sensitive to the dopaminergic state. A recent addiction animal model demonstrated that low-frequency stimulation of the nucleus accumbens reversed cocaine-evoked plasticity [157]. In clinical research, DTI and fMRI before DBS and after 5 months of DBS (at this time, the patient's DBS system was extracted because of other problems) indicated shifted images toward more typical images of a normal healthy control [11]. Although this study comprises a single human report, these changes induced by DBS will be reproducible in the future. A substantial number of PET studies have previously demonstrated that DBS in OCD, dystonia, depression or PD reversed the metabolic activity or cerebral blood flow toward the normal baseline [158–164].

The neuroprotective or neuroregenerative effects of DBS remain uncertain. However, there are limited reports regarding the neuroprotective effects of DBS. A Parkinsonian rat model subjected to STN DBS or STN lesioning exhibited an improvement in the survival of substantia nigra pars compacta neurons [165–167]. It has been suggested that this effect was result of a reduction of glutamatergic excitation from STN hyperactivity [168]. STN DBS has been demonstrated to induce the neuroprotective growth factor brain-derived neurotrophic factor (BDNF) in the substantia nigra, GPi, and primary motor cortex [169]. Furthermore, GPi DBS altered glial-derived neurotrophic factor (GDNF) expression in the basal ganglia (BG) in an animal model [170]. The potential neuroprotective effects of DBS remain under vigorous investigation.

4. Brain connectivity and DBS

4.1. Modalities used to investigate brain connectivity

Researchers have used several modalities to investigate brain connectivity. Classical imaging modalities have demonstrated structural connectivity that indicates the morphometric properties of the brain, such as the volume of grey matter and connecting fibers through white mater. High-resolution T1-weighted MRI has been used to investigate structural connectivity via voxel-based morphometry [171]. DTI comprises a well-known method to identify brain structures by measuring the directional diffusion of water molecules. Recently, diffusion-weighted imaging (DWI) and fiber tractography have been used to assess the white mater microstructure and pathways of the whole brain [172, 173]. DWI uses the passive diffusion of water molecules to infer the properties of the surrounding tissue.

Functional imaging modalities include fMRI, PET, and SPECT, which indicate dynamic changes in hemodynamics or metabolism in the brain and are related to neural activity. These modalities have provided a window into the global and long-term changes in network activity as a result of DBS [174, 175]. They are unique to obtain system-level data in brain network activity; however, the data represent the indirect effects of neural activities and changes in afferent input to the activated region, not output [176]. Functional connectivity has been defined as the temporal correlations between spatially remote neurophysiological events [177, 178]. One of the prevalent modalities used to assess functional connectivity is EEG, which has been used to assess the brain electrical activities using electrodes placed on the scalp. The high temporal resolution of EEG provided the benefit of estimating the changes in functional network connectivity [8]. MEG is also an option to evaluate the electrical activities of the brain. EEG and MEG data have provided valuable information regarding diseased brains, such as in Alzheimer's disease, epilepsy, schizophrenia, Parkinson's disease, and other neurological conditions [9, 179–182].

Structural and functional imaging modalities have their own specific spatial and temporal scales, and they are primarily evaluated independently. Recently, a multimodal approach has been attempted to better understand the structure–function associations. EEG–fMRI, EEG–DTI, fMRI–DTI, and other fusion applications have been reported [183].

4.2. Brain connectivity

The most common clinical form of DBS comprises the stimulation of the subthalamic region for PD patients. Currently, the most common research form of functional connectivity is based on studies of the BG stimulation. The author would like to briefly review the BG anatomy and neuromodulation of DBS via BG stimulation.

Four core nuclei compose the BG, which include the striatum (caudate nucleus and putamen), globus pallidus (internus (GPi) and externus (GPe)), substantia nigra (pars compacta (SNc) and pars reticulate (SNr)), and the STN [184–186]. The striatum and the STN receive inputs from the cortex, and the GPi and SNr provide BG output to the thalamus and brainstem. Striatal neurons comprise the direct (D1) and indirect (D2) pathways. The direct pathway is a monosynaptic inhibitory pathway (GABA-ergic), and the indirect pathway is a polysynaptic and net excitatory pathway that involves the GPe and STN. Additional input originates from the thalamic intralaminar nuclei. GABA-ergic projections from the striatum inhibit thalamocortical projection neurons on the ventral anterior, ventrolateral, and intralaminar nuclei of the thalamus and brain stem neurons. Indirect projections from the striatum result in a net excitatory effect on the GPi and SNr, whereas direct projections exert an inhibitory effect on these output nuclei (**Figure 2**).

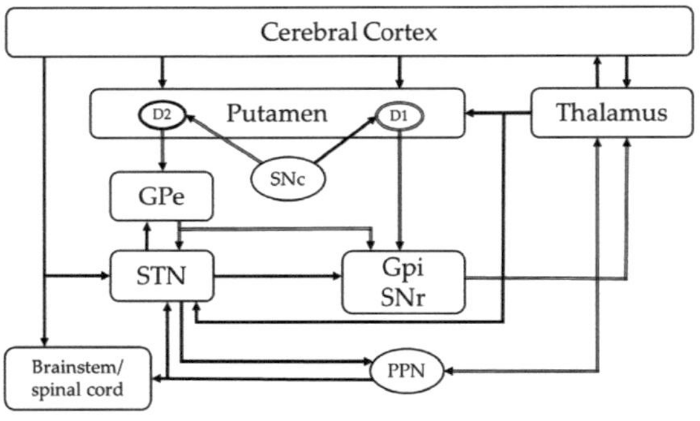

Figure 2. Connections of basal ganglia motor circuit. Solid arrows indicate excitatory (glutamatergic neurons) and double stranded arrows indicate inhibitory (GABA-ergic neurons). GPe, globus pallidus externus; GPi, globus pallidus internus; SNc, substantia nigra pars compacta; SNr, substantia nigra pars reticulata; STN, subthalamic nucleus; PPN, pedunculopontine nucleus

There has been an increasing interest in the use of functional imaging to investigate the global brain effects of STN DBS in PD patients [187–191]. The functional imaging of PD patients indicated hypermetabolism in the pons, globus pallidus, and thalamus and hypometabolism in the premotor cortex, supplementary motor area, and parietal association area [192, 193]. In an fMRI study of STN DBS patients, activations were identified in a broad sensorimotor network, including the sensorimotor, supplementary motor and cingulate cortices, insula, caudate nucleus, pedunculopontine nucleus (PPN), and cerebellum [175].

Experimental recordings have also demonstrated the phenomena of functional connectivity. An animal extracellular recording demonstrated increased neuronal activity in the GPi during clinically effective STN DBS, which is consistent with an increase in excitatory output from the STN [194]. Intracellular recording in rodents demonstrated STN DBS elicited antidromic action potentials to the cortex [195]. Microdialysis performed in humans during the implantation of a clinically effective DBS system resulted in increased extracellular cyclic guanosine 3′: 5′-cyclic monophosphate (cGMP) concentrations in the putamen, GPi, and SNr [196–199]. Extracellular cGMP is an indirect marker of local glutamatergic synaptic input, which is consistent with stimulation increasing STN output [200].

In a case of dystonia, the connection of the GPi to the ventral oralis posterior nucleus (Vop) of the thalamus was reported via microelectrode monitoring of the Vop during GPi DBS for generalized dystonia [201]. In this report, GPi stimulation provoked the activation of axons to the Vop and the antidromic activation of Vop axons; however, this was a case report.

5. Future of DBS

DBS is a well-established therapeutic option for various conditions. The surgical procedures are standardized but differ across centers. The complications are acceptable based on previous, well-designed studies. However, new targets and clinical indications are continuously emerging, and vigorous investigations are ongoing. The technical advancement of implantable devices is amazingly rapid. The author has confidence that a closed circuit system, as well as a more advanced technological system, will be invented in the near future.

To date, DBS is not only a clinical treatment option but is an amazingly powerful research tool; however, its mechanism and effects on the brain network continue to be investigated. Functional connectivity within the brain may be validated by the use of multimodal approaches using various tools.

Acknowledgements

This work was supported by a grant from research year of Inje University in 2015.

Author details

Hae Yu Kim

Address all correspondence to: hykim080356@gmail.com

Stereotactic & Functional Section, Department of Neurosurgery, Haeundae Paik Hospital, Inje University College of Medicine, Busan, South Korea

References

[1] Benabid AL, Pollak P, Louveau A, Henry S, de Rougemont J. Combined (thalamotomy and stimulation) stereotactic surgery of the VIM thalamic nucleus for bilateral Parkinson disease. *Appl Neurophysiol*. 1987; 50(1–6):344–346.

[2] Benabid A, Chabardes S, Torres N, Piallat B, Krack P, Fraix V, et al. Functional neurosurgery for movement disorders: a historical perspective. *Prog Brain Res*. 2009; 175:379–391. DOI: 10.1016/S0079-6123(09)17525-8.

[3] McIntyre C, Hahn P. Network perspectives on the mechanisms of deep brain stimulation. *Neurobiol Dis*. 2010; 38(3):329–337. DOI: 10.1016/j.nbd.2009.09.022.

[4] Okun M. Deep-brain stimulation—entering the era of human neural-network modulation. *N Engl J Med*. 2014; 371(15):1369–1373. DOI: 10.1056/NEJMp1408779.

[5] Kahan J, Urner M, Moran R, Flandin G, Marreiros A, Mancini L, et al. Resting state functional MRI in Parkinson's disease: the impact of deep brain stimulation on "effective" connectivity. *Brain*. 2014; 137(4):1130–1144. DOI: 10.1093/brain/awu027.

[6] Buchanan CR, Pernet CR, Gorgolewski KJ, Storkey AJ, Bastin ME. Test–retest reliability of structural brain networks from diffusion MRI. *Neuroimage*. 2014; 86:231–243.

[7] Gudayol Ferré E, Peró Cebollero M, González Garrido A, Guàrdia Olmos J. Changes in brain connectivity related to the treatment of depression measured through fMRI: a systematic review. *Front Hum Neurosci*. 2015; 9:582. DOI: 10.3389/fnhum.2015.00582.

[8] Horn A, Ostwald D, Reisert M, Blankenburg F. The structural-functional connectome and the default mode network of the human brain. *Neuroimage*. 2014; 102 Pt 1:142–151. DOI: 10.1016/j.neuroimage.2013.09.069.

[9] van Diessen E, Numan T, van Dellen E, van der Kooi AW, Boersma M, Hofman D, et al. Opportunities and methodological challenges in EEG and MEG resting state functional brain network research. *Clin Neurophysiol*. 2015; 126(8):1468–1481. DOI: 10.1016/j.clinph.2014.11.018.

[10] van Straaten ECW, Stam C. Structure out of chaos: functional brain network analysis with EEG, MEG, and functional MRI. *Eur Neuropsychopharmacol*. 2013; 23(1):7–18. DOI: 10.1016/j.euroneuro.2012.10.010.

[11] van Hartevelt T, Cabral J, Deco G, Møller A, Green A, Aziz T, et al. Neural plasticity in human brain connectivity: the effects of long term deep brain stimulation of the subthalamic nucleus in Parkinson's disease. *PLoS ONE*. 2014; 9(1):e86496. DOI: 10.1371/journal.pone.0086496.

[12] Fritsch G, Hitzig E. Electric excitability of the cerebrum. Archives für Anatomie Physiologie und Wissenshaftlicke Medicin, 300–332. Trans, by G.von Bonin (1960), in Some Papers on The Cerebral Cortex. 1870:73–96.

[13] Vilensky J, Gilman S. Horsley was the first to use electrical stimulation of the human cerebral cortex intraoperatively. *Surg Neurol*. 2002; 58(6):425–426. DOI: 10.1016/S0090-3019(02)00920-5.

[14] Spiegel EA, Wycis HT, Marks M, Lee AJ. Stereotaxic apparatus for operations on the human brain. *Science*. 1947; 106(2754):349–350. DOI: 10.1126/science.106.2754.349.

[15] Compston A. The structure and functions of the cerebellum examined by a new method. By Sir Victor Horsley, FRS, FRCS and RH Clarke, MA, MB. *Brain*. 1908; 31:45–124.

[16] Hassler R, Riechert T, Mundinger F, Umbach W, Ganglberger JA. Physiological observations in stereotaxic operations in extrapyramidal motor disturbances. *Brain*. 1960; 83:337–350. DOI: 10.1093/brain/83.2.337.

[17] Alberts WW, Feinstein B, Levin G, Wright EW. Electrical stimulation of therapeutic targets in waking dyskinetic patients. *Electroencephalogr Clin Neurophysiol*. 1966; 20(6): 559–566. DOI: 10.1016/0013-4694(66)90020-4.

[18] Delgado JM, Hamlin H, Chapman WP. Technique of intracranial electrode implacement for recording and stimulation and its possible therapeutic value in psychotic patients. *Stereotact Funct Neurosurg*. 1952; 12(5–6):315–319.

[19] Heath RG. Depth recording and stimulation studies in patients. In: Winter A, editor. *The Surgical Control of Behavior*. Springfield, IL: Charles C Thomas; 1971. p. 21–37.

[20] Gildenberg P. Evolution of neuromodulation. *Stereotact Funct Neurosurg*. 2005; 83(2–3): 71–79. DOI: 10.1159/000086865.

[21] Shealy CN, Mortimer JT, Reswick JB. Electrical inhibition of pain by stimulation of the dorsal columns: preliminary clinical report. *Anesth Analg*. 1967; 46(4):489–491. DOI: 10.1213/00000539-196707000-00025.

[22] Cooper IS, Riklan M, Amin I, Waltz JM, Cullinan T. Chronic cerebellar stimulation in cerebral palsy. *Neurology*. 1976; 26(8):744–753. DOI: 10.1212/WNL.26.8.744.

[23] Cooper IS, Amin I, Riklan M, Waltz JM, Poon TP. Chronic cerebellar stimulation in epilepsy. Clinical and anatomical studies. *Arch Neurol*. 1976; 33(8):559–570. DOI: 10.1001/archneur.1976.00500080037006.

[24] Hosobuchi Y, Adams JE, Rutkin B. Chronic thalamic stimulation for the control of facial anesthesia dolorosa. *Arch Neurol*. 1973; 29(3):158–161. DOI: 10.1001/archneur.1973.00490270040005.

[25] Tóth S, Tomka I. Responses of the human thalamus and pallidum to high frequency stimulations. *Confin Neurol*. 1968; 30(1):17–40. DOI: 10.1159/000103517.

[26] Brice J, McLellan L. Suppression of intention tremor by contingent deep-brain stimulation. Lancet. 1980; 1(8180):1221–1222. DOI: 10.1016/S0140-6736(80)91680-3.

[27] Siegfried J. Effect of stimulation of the sensory nucleus of the thalamus on dyskinesia and spasticity. *Rev Neurol (Paris)*. 1986; 142(4):380–383.

[28] Laitinen LV, Bergenheim AT, Hariz MI. Leksell's posteroventral pallidotomy in the treatment of Parkinson's disease. *J Neurosurg*. 1992; 76(1):53–61. DOI: 10.3171/jns.1992.76.1.0053.

[29] Siegfried J, Lippitz B. Chronic electrical stimulation of the VL-VPL complex and of the pallidum in the treatment of movement disorders: personal experience since 1982. *Stereotact Funct Neurosurg*. 1994; 62(1–4):71–75. DOI: 10.1159/000098599.

[30] Lozano A. Deep brain stimulation: challenges to integrating stimulation technology with human neurobiology, neuroplasticity, and neural repair. *J Rehabil Res Dev*. 2001; 38(6):x–xix.

[31] Ashby P, Strafella A, Dostrovsky JO, Lozano A, Lang AE. Immediate motor effects of stimulation through electrodes implanted in the human globus pallidus. *Stereotact Funct Neurosurg*. 1998; 70(1):1–18. DOI: 10.1159/000029593.

[32] Benabid AL, Pollak P, Gross C, Hoffmann D, Benazzouz A, Gao DM, et al. Acute and long-term effects of subthalamic nucleus stimulation in Parkinson's disease. *Stereotact Funct Neurosurg*. 1994; 62(1–4):76–84. DOI: 10.1159/000098600.

[33] Hariz M. Twenty-five years of deep brain stimulation: celebrations and apprehensions. *Mov Disord*. 2012; 27(7):930–933. DOI: 10.1002/mds.25007.

[34] Fukaya C, Yamamoto T. Deep brain stimulation for Parkinson's disease: recent trends and future direction. *Neurol Med Chir* (Tokyo). 2015; 55(5):422–431. DOI: 10.2176/nmc.ra.2014-0446.

[35] St George RJ, Nutt JG, Burchiel KJ, Horak FB. A meta-regression of the long-term effects of deep brain stimulation on balance and gait in PD. *Neurology*. 2010; 75(14):1292–1299. DOI: 10.1212/WNL.0b013e3181f61329.

[36] Odekerken VJJ, van Laar T, Staal M, Mosch A, Hoffmann CFE, Nijssen PCG, et al. Subthalamic nucleus versus globus pallidus bilateral deep brain stimulation for

advanced Parkinson's disease (NSTAPS study): a randomised controlled trial. *Lancet Neurol.* 2013; 12(1):37–44. DOI: 10.1016/S1474-4422(12)70264-8.

[37] Weaver F, Follett K, Stern M, Luo P, Harris C, Hur K, et al. Randomized trial of deep brain stimulation for Parkinson disease: thirty-six-month outcomes. *Neurology.* 2012; 79(1):55–65. DOI: 10.1212/WNL.0b013e31825dcdc1.

[38] Follett K, Weaver F, Stern M, Hur K, Harris C, Luo P, et al. Pallidal versus subthalamic deep-brain stimulation for Parkinson's disease. *N Engl J Med.* 2010; 362(22):2077–2091. DOI: 10.1056/NEJMoa0907083.

[39] Bot M, van den Munckhof P, Bakay R, Sierens D, Stebbins G, Verhagen Metman L. Analysis of stereotactic accuracy in patients undergoing deep brain stimulation using nexframe and the leksell frame. *Stereotact Funct Neurosurg.* 2015; 93(5):316–325. DOI: 10.1159/000375178.

[40] Sharma M, Rhiew R, Deogaonkar M, Rezai A, Boulis N. Accuracy and precision of targeting using frameless stereotactic system in deep brain stimulator implantation surgery. *Neurol India.* 2014; 62(5):503–509. DOI: 10.4103/0028-3886.144442.

[41] Fukaya C, Sumi K, Otaka T, Obuchi T, Kano T, Kobayashi K, et al. Nexframe frameless stereotaxy with multitract microrecording: accuracy evaluated by frame-based stereotactic X-ray. *Stereotact Funct Neurosurg.* 2010; 88(3):163–168. DOI: 10.1159/000313868.

[42] Kocabicak E, Temel Y. Deep brain stimulation of the subthalamic nucleus in Parkinson's disease: surgical technique, tips, tricks and complications. *Clin Neurol Neurosurg.* 2013; 115(11):2318–2323. DOI: 10.1016/j.clineuro.2013.08.020.

[43] Tanei T, Kajita Y, Kaneoke Y, Takebayashi S, Nakatsubo D, Wakabayashi T. Staged bilateral deep brain stimulation of the subthalamic nucleus for the treatment of Parkinson's disease. *Acta Neurochir* (Wien). 2009; 151(6):589–594. DOI: 10.1007/s00701-009-0293-6.

[44] Reck C, Maarouf M, Wojtecki L, Groiss S, Florin E, Sturm V, et al. Clinical outcome of subthalamic stimulation in Parkinson's disease is improved by intraoperative multiple trajectories microelectrode recording. *J Neurol Surg A Cent Eur Neurosurg.* 2012; 73(6): 377–386. DOI: 10.1055/s-0032-1326957.

[45] Kim HY, Lee S, Jin SJ, Kim JS, Jeon KD. Reliability of stereotactic coordinates of 1.5-T and 3-T MRI in radiosurgery and functional neurosurgery. *J Korean Neurosurg Soc.* 2014; 55(3):136–141. DOI: 10.3340/jkns.2014.55.3.136.

[46] Park YS, Kang JH, Kim HY, Kang DW, Chang WS, Kim JP, et al. A combination procedure with double C-shaped skin incision and dual-floor burr hole method to prevent skin erosion on the scalp and reduce postoperative skin complications in deep brain stimulation. *Stereotact Funct Neurosurg.* 2011; 89(3):178–184. DOI: 10.1159/000324903.

[47] Petersen E, Holl E, Martinez Torres I, Foltynie T, Limousin P, Hariz M, et al. Minimizing brain shift in stereotactic functional neurosurgery. *Neurosurgery*. 2010; 67(3 Suppl Operative):ons213–ons221; discussion on 221. DOI: 10.1227/01.NEU.0000380991.23444.08.

[48] Chang WS, Kim HY, Kim JP, Park YS, Chung SS, Chang JW. Bilateral subthalamic deep brain stimulation using single track microelectrode recording. *Acta Neurochir* (Wien). 2011; 153(5):1087–1095. DOI: 10.1007/s00701-011-0953-1.

[49] Hodaie M, Wennberg R, Dostrovsky J, Lozano A. Chronic anterior thalamus stimulation for intractable epilepsy. *Epilepsia*. 2002; 43(6):603–608. DOI: 10.1046/j.1528-1157.2002.26001.x.

[50] Kerrigan J, Litt B, Fisher R, Cranstoun S, French J, Blum D, et al. Electrical stimulation of the anterior nucleus of the thalamus for the treatment of intractable epilepsy. *Epilepsia*. 2004; 45(4):346–354. DOI: 10.1111/j.0013-9580.2004.01304.x.

[51] Machado A, Rezai A, Kopell B, Gross R, Sharan A, Benabid A. Deep brain stimulation for Parkinson's disease: surgical technique and perioperative management. *Mov Disord*. 2006; 21 Suppl 14:S247-S258. DOI: 10.1002/mds.20959.

[52] Sadeghi Y, Pralong E, Knebel J, Vingerhoets F, Pollo C, Levivier M, et al. Bilateral deep brain stimulation: the placement of the second electrode is not necessarily less accurate than that of the first one. *Stereotact Funct Neurosurg*. 2015; 93(3):160–167. DOI: 10.1159/000368439.

[53] Petraglia F, Farber SH, Han J, Verla T, Gallis J, Lokhnygina Y, et al. Comparison of bilateral vs. staged unilateral deep brain stimulation (dbs) in Parkinson's disease in patients under 70 years of age. *Neuromodulation*. 2016; 19(1):31–37. DOI: 10.1111/ner.12351.

[54] Papapetropoulos S, Salcedo A, Singer C, Gallo B, Jagid J. Staged unilateral or bilateral STN-DBS? *Mov Disord*. 2008; 23(5):775. DOI: 10.1002/mds.21916.

[55] Samii A, Kelly V, Slimp J, Shumway Cook A, Goodkin R. Staged unilateral versus bilateral subthalamic nucleus stimulator implantation in Parkinson disease. *Mov Disord*. 2007; 22(10):1476–1481. DOI: 10.1002/mds.21554.

[56] Abosch A, Timmermann L, Bartley S, Rietkerk H, Whiting D, Connolly P, et al. An international survey of deep brain stimulation procedural steps. *Stereotact Funct Neurosurg*. 2013; 91(1):1–11. DOI: 10.1159/000343207.

[57] Carlson J, Neumiller J, Swain LDW, Mark J, McLeod P, Hirschauer J. Postoperative delirium in Parkinson's disease patients following deep brain stimulation surgery. *J Clin Neurosci*. 2014; 21(7):1192–1195. DOI: 10.1016/j.jocn.2013.12.007.

[58] Zhang K, Bhatia S, Oh M, Cohen D, Angle C, Whiting D. Long-term results of thalamic deep brain stimulation for essential tremor. *J Neurosurg*. 2010; 112(6):1271–1276. DOI: 10.3171/2009.10.JNS09371.

[59] Lyons K, Pahwa R. Deep brain stimulation and essential tremor. *J Clin Neurophysiol.* 2004; 21(1):2–5. DOI: 10.1097/00004691-200401000-00002.

[60] Baizabal Carvallo J, Kagnoff M, Jimenez Shahed J, Fekete R, Jankovic J. The safety and efficacy of thalamic deep brain stimulation in essential tremor: 10 years and beyond. *J Neurol Neurosurg Psychiatr*. 2014; 85(5):567–572. DOI: 10.1136/jnnp-2013-304943.

[61] Pilitsis J, Metman L, Toleikis J, Hughes L, Sani S, Bakay RAE. Factors involved in long-term efficacy of deep brain stimulation of the thalamus for essential tremor. *J Neurosurg*. 2008; 109(4):640–646. DOI: 10.3171/JNS/2008/109/10/0640.

[62] Blomstedt P, Hariz G, Hariz MI, Koskinen LD. Thalamic deep brain stimulation in the treatment of essential tremor: a long-term follow-up. *Br J Neurosurg*. 2007; 21(5):504–509. DOI: 10.1080/02688690701552278.

[63] Sydow O, Thobois S, Alesch F, Speelman JD. Multicentre European study of thalamic stimulation in essential tremor: a six year follow up. *J Neurol Neurosurg Psychiatr*. 2003; 74(10):1387–1391. DOI: 10.1136/jnnp.74.10.1387.

[64] Limousin P, Speelman JD, Gielen F, Janssens M. Multicentre European study of thalamic stimulation in parkinsonian and essential tremor. *J Neurol Neurosurg Psychiatr*. 1999; 66(3):289–296. DOI: 10.1136/jnnp.66.3.289.

[65] Rehncrona S, Johnels B, Widner H, Törnqvist A, Hariz M, Sydow O. Long-term efficacy of thalamic deep brain stimulation for tremor: double-blind assessments. *Mov Disord*. 2003; 18(2):163–170. DOI: 10.1002/mds.10309.

[66] Limousin P, Speelman JD, Gielen F, Janssens M. Multicentre European study of thalamic stimulation in parkinsonian and essential tremor. *J Neurol Neurosurg Psychiatr*. 1999; 66(3):289–296. DOI: 10.1136/jnnp.66.3.289.

[67] Obwegeser AA, Uitti RJ, Turk MF, Strongosky AJ, Wharen RE. Thalamic stimulation for the treatment of midline tremors in essential tremor patients. *Neurology*. 2000; 54(12): 2342–2344. DOI: 10.1212/WNL.54.12.2342.

[68] Koller WC, Lyons KE, Wilkinson SB, Troster AI, Pahwa R. Long-term safety and efficacy of unilateral deep brain stimulation of the thalamus in essential tremor. *Mov Disord*. 2001; 16(3):464–468. DOI: 10.1002/mds.1089.

[69] Benabid AL, Pollak P, Gao D, Hoffmann D, Limousin P, Gay E, et al. Chronic electrical stimulation of the ventralis intermedius nucleus of the thalamus as a treatment of movement disorders. *J Neurosurg*. 1996; 84(2):203–214. DOI: 10.3171/jns.1996.84.2.0203.

[70] Lang A. Assessment of Parkinson's disease. In: Munsat TL, editor. *Quantification of Neurological Deficit*. Stonehame, MA: Butterworths; 1989. p. 285–309.

[71] Hoehn MM, Yahr MD. Parkinsonism: onset, progression, and mortality. 1967. *Neurology*. 2001; 57(10 Suppl 3):S11-S26.

[72] Peto V, Jenkinson C, Fitzpatrick R, Greenhall R. The development and validation of a short measure of functioning and well being for individuals with Parkinson's disease. *Qual Life Res*. 1995; 4(3):241–248. DOI: 10.1007/BF02260863.

[73] Jankovic J, Poewe W. Therapies in Parkinson's disease. *Curr Opin Neurol*. 2012; 25(4): 433–447. DOI: 10.1097/WCO.0b013e3283542fc2.

[74] Schuepbach W, Rau J, Knudsen K, Volkmann J, Krack P, Timmermann L, et al. Neurostimulation for Parkinson's disease with early motor complications. *N Engl J Med*. 2013; 368(7):610–622.

[75] Deuschl G, Schade Brittinger C, Krack P, Volkmann J, Schäfer H, Bötzel K, et al. A randomized trial of deep-brain stimulation for Parkinson's disease. *N Engl J Med*. 2006; 355(9):896–908. DOI: 10.1056/NEJMoa060281.

[76] Williams A, Gill S, Varma T, Jenkinson C, Quinn N, Mitchell R, et al. Deep brain stimulation plus best medical therapy versus best medical therapy alone for advanced Parkinson's disease (PD SURG trial): a randomised, open-label trial. *Lancet Neurol*. 2010; 9(6):581–591. DOI: 10.1016/S1474-4422(10)70093-4.

[77] Fasano A, Romito L, Daniele A, Piano C, Zinno M, Bentivoglio A, et al. Motor and cognitive outcome in patients with Parkinson's disease 8 years after subthalamic implants. *Brain*. 2010; 133(9):2664–2676. DOI: 10.1093/brain/awq221.

[78] Castrioto A, Lozano A, Poon Y, Lang A, Fallis M, Moro E. Ten-year outcome of subthalamic stimulation in Parkinson disease: a blinded evaluation. *Arch Neurol*. 2011; 68(12):1550–1556. DOI: 10.1001/archneurol.2011.182.

[79] Zibetti M, Merola A, Rizzi L, Ricchi V, Angrisano S, Azzaro C, et al. Beyond nine years of continuous subthalamic nucleus deep brain stimulation in Parkinson's disease. *Mov Disord*. 2011; 26(13):2327–2334. DOI: 10.1002/mds.23903.

[80] Burke RE, Fahn S, Marsden CD, Bressman SB, Moskowitz C, Friedman J. Validity and reliability of a rating scale for the primary torsion dystonias. *Neurology*. 1985; 35(1):73–77. DOI: 10.1212/WNL.35.1.73.

[81] Boyce M, Canning C, Mahant N, Morris J, Latimer J, Fung VSC. The Toronto Western Spasmodic Torticollis Rating Scale: reliability in neurologists and physiotherapists. *Parkinsonism Relat Disord*. 2012; 18(5):635–637. DOI: 10.1016/j.parkreldis.2012.02.007.

[82] Vercueil L, Pollak P, Fraix V, Caputo E, Moro E, Benazzouz A, et al. Deep brain stimulation in the treatment of severe dystonia. *J Neurol*. 2001; 248(8):695–700. DOI: 10.1007/s004150170116.

[83] Coubes P, Cif L, El Fertit H, Hemm S, Vayssiere N, Serrat S, et al. Electrical stimulation of the globus pallidus internus in patients with primary generalized dystonia: long-term results. *J Neurosurg*. 2004; 101(2):189–194. DOI: 10.3171/jns.2004.101.2.0189.

[84] Cif L, El Fertit H, Vayssiere N, Hemm S, Hardouin E, Gannau A, et al. Treatment of dystonic syndromes by chronic electrical stimulation of the internal globus pallidus. *J Neurosurg Sci*. 2003; 47(1):52–55.

[85] Vidailhet M, Vercueil L, Houeto J, Krystkowiak P, Benabid A, Cornu P, et al. Bilateral deep-brain stimulation of the globus pallidus in primary generalized dystonia. *N Engl J Med*. 2005; 352(5):459–467. DOI: 10.1056/NEJMoa042187.

[86] Kupsch A, Benecke R, Trottenberg T, Schneider G, Poewe W, Eisner W, et al. Pallidal deep-brain stimulation in primary generalized or segmental dystonia. *N Engl J Med*. 2006; 355(19):1978–1990. DOI: 10.1056/NEJMoa063618.

[87] Valldeoriola F, Regidor I, Mínguez Castellanos A, Lezcano E, García Ruiz P, Rojo A, et al. Efficacy and safety of pallidal stimulation in primary dystonia: results of the Spanish multicentric study. *J Neurol Neurosurg Psychiatr*. 2010; 81(1):65–69. DOI: 10.1136/jnnp.2009.174342.

[88] Damier P, Thobois S, Witjas T, Cuny E, Derost P, Raoul S, et al. Bilateral deep brain stimulation of the globus pallidus to treat tardive dyskinesia. *Arch Gen Psychiatry*. 2007; 64(2):170–176. DOI: 10.1001/archpsyc.64.2.170.

[89] Chang E, Schrock L, Starr P, Ostrem J. Long-term benefit sustained after bilateral pallidal deep brain stimulation in patients with refractory tardive dystonia. *Stereotact Funct Neurosurg*. 2010; 88(5):304–310. DOI: 10.1159/000316763.

[90] Skogseid IM, Ramm Pettersen J, Volkmann J, Kerty E, Dietrichs E, Røste GK. Good long-term efficacy of pallidal stimulation in cervical dystonia: a prospective, observer-blinded study. *Eur J Neurol*. 2012; 19(4):610–615. DOI: 10.1111/j.1468-1331.2011.03591.x.

[91] Hung SW, Hamani C, Lozano AM, Poon YW, Piboolnurak P, Miyasaki JM, et al. Long-term outcome of bilateral pallidal deep brain stimulation for primary cervical dystonia. *Neurology*. 2007; 68(6):457–459. DOI: 10.1212/01.wnl.0000252932.71306.89.

[92] Kiss ZHT, Doig Beyaert K, Eliasziw M, Tsui J, Haffenden A, Suchowersky O. The Canadian multicentre study of deep brain stimulation for cervical dystonia. *Brain*. 2007; 130(11):2879–2886. DOI: 10.1093/brain/awm229.

[93] Walsh R, Sidiropoulos C, Lozano A, Hodaie M, Poon Y, Fallis M, et al. Bilateral pallidal stimulation in cervical dystonia: blinded evidence of benefit beyond 5 years. *Brain*. 2013; 136(3):761–769. DOI: 10.1093/brain/awt009.

[94] Kleiner Fisman G, Herzog J, Fisman D, Tamma F, Lyons K, Pahwa R, et al. Subthalamic nucleus deep brain stimulation: summary and meta-analysis of outcomes. *Mov Disord*. 2006; 21 Suppl 14:S290-S304. DOI: 10.1002/mds.20962.

[95] Binder D, Rau G, Starr P. Risk factors for hemorrhage during microelectrode-guided deep brain stimulator implantation for movement disorders. *Neurosurgery*. 2005; 56(4): 722–732; discussion 722. DOI: 10.1227/01.NEU.0000156473.57196.7E.

[96] Binder D, Rau G, Starr P. Hemorrhagic complications of microelectrode-guided deep brain stimulation. Stereotact Funct Neurosurg. 2003; 80(1–4):28–31. DOI: 10.1159/000075156.

[97] Lyons K, Wilkinson S, Overman J, Pahwa R. Surgical and hardware complications of subthalamic stimulation: a series of 160 procedures. *Neurology*. 2004; 63(4):612–616. DOI: 10.1212/01.WNL.0000134650.91974.1A.

[98] Kenney C, Simpson R, Hunter C, Ondo W, Almaguer M, Davidson A, et al. Short-term and long-term safety of deep brain stimulation in the treatment of movement disorders. *J Neurosurg*. 2007; 106(4):621–625. DOI: 10.3171/jns.2007.106.4.621.

[99] Hamani C, Lozano A. Hardware-related complications of deep brain stimulation: a review of the published literature. *Stereotact Funct Neurosurg*. 2006; 84(5–6):248–251. DOI: 10.1159/000096499.

[100] Kim HY, Chang WS, Kang DW, Sohn YH, Lee MS, Chang JW. Factors related to outcomes of subthalamic deep brain stimulation in Parkinson's disease. J *Korean Neurosurg Soc*. 2013; 54(2):118–124. DOI: 10.3340/jkns.2013.54.2.118.

[101] Temel Y, Wilbrink P, Duits A, Boon P, Tromp S, Ackermans L, et al. Single electrode and multiple electrode guided electrical stimulation of the subthalamic nucleus in advanced Parkinson's disease. *Neurosurgery*. 2007; 61(5 Suppl 2):346–355; discussion 355. DOI: 10.1227/01.neu.0000303993.82149.98.

[102] Xiaowu H, Xiufeng J, Xiaoping Z, Bin H, Laixing W, Yiqun C, et al. Risks of intracranial hemorrhage in patients with Parkinson's disease receiving deep brain stimulation and ablation. *Parkinsonism Relat Disord*. 2010; 16(2):96–100. DOI: 10.1016/j.parkreldis.2009.07.013.

[103] Morishita T, Okun M, Burdick A, Jacobson C, Foote K. Cerebral venous infarction: a potentially avoidable complication of deep brain stimulation surgery. *Neuromodulation*. 2013; 16(5):407–413; discussion 413. DOI: 10.1111/ner.12052.

[104] Machado A, Deogaonkar M, Cooper S. Deep brain stimulation for movement disorders: patient selection and technical options. *Cleve Clin J Med*. 2012; 79 Suppl 2:S19-S24. DOI: 10.3949/ccjm.79.s2a.04.

[105] Kang DW, Kim HY, Chang JW. Cerebral ischemia related to globus pallidus internus stimulation for cervical dystonia. *Stereotact Funct Neurosurg*. 2011; 89(4):201–204. DOI: 10.1159/000325655.

[106] Novak K, Nenonene E, Bernstein L, Vergenz S, Medalle G, Prager J, et al. Two cases of ischemia associated with subthalamic nucleus stimulator implantation for advanced Parkinson's disease. *Mov Disord*. 2006; 21(9):1477–1483. DOI: 10.1002/mds.20947.

[107] Okun M, Tagliati M, Pourfar M, Fernandez H, Rodriguez R, Alterman R, et al. Management of referred deep brain stimulation failures: a retrospective analysis from 2

movement disorders centers. *Arch Neurol*. 2005; 62(8):1250–1255. DOI: 10.1001/archneur.62.8.noc40425.

[108] Blomstedt P, Hariz MI. Hardware-related complications of deep brain stimulation: a ten year experience. *Acta Neurochir (Wien)*. 2005; 147(10):1061–1064; discussion 1064. DOI: 10.1007/s00701-005-0576-5.

[109] Hamel W, Schrader B, Weinert D, Herzog J, Müller D, Deuschl G, et al. Technical complication in deep brain stimulation. *Zentralbl Neurochir*. 2002; 63(3):124–127. DOI: 10.1055/s-2002-35822.

[110] Hariz MI, Fodstad H. Do microelectrode techniques increase accuracy or decrease risks in pallidotomy and deep brain stimulation? A critical review of the literature. *Stereotact Funct Neurosurg*. 1999; 72(2–4):157–169. DOI: 10.1159/000029720.

[111] Deep-Brain Stimulation for Parkinson's Disease Study Group. Deep-brain stimulation of the subthalamic nucleus or the pars interna of the globus pallidus in Parkinson's disease. *N Engl J Med*. 2001; 345(13):956–963. DOI: 10.1056/NEJMoa000827.

[112] Beric A, Kelly PJ, Rezai A, Sterio D, Mogilner A, Zonenshayn M, et al. Complications of deep brain stimulation surgery. *Stereotact Funct Neurosurg*. 2001; 77(1–4):73–78. DOI: 10.1159/000064600.

[113] Oh M, Abosch A, Kim S, Lang A, Lozano A. Long-term hardware-related complications of deep brain stimulation. *Neurosurgery*. 2002; 50(6):1268–1274; discussion 1274.

[114] Voges J, Waerzeggers Y, Maarouf M, Lehrke R, Koulousakis A, Lenartz D, et al. Deep-brain stimulation: long-term analysis of complications caused by hardware and surgery--experiences from a single centre. *J Neurol Neurosurg Psychiatr*. 2006; 77(7):868–872. DOI: 10.1136/jnnp.2005.081232.

[115] Vesper J, Haak S, Ostertag C, Nikkhah G. Subthalamic nucleus deep brain stimulation in elderly patients--analysis of outcome and complications. *BMC Neurol*. 2007; 7:7. DOI: 10.1186/1471-2377-7-7.

[116] Blomstedt P, Hariz M. Are complications less common in deep brain stimulation than in ablative procedures for movement disorders? *Stereotact Funct Neurosurg*. 2006; 84(2–3):72–81. DOI: 10.1159/000094035.

[117] Coubes P, Vayssiere N, El Fertit H, Hemm S, Cif L, Kienlen J, et al. Deep brain stimulation for dystonia. Surgical technique. *Stereotact Funct Neurosurg*. 2002; 78(3–4):183–191. DOI: 10.1159/000068962.

[118] Deuschl G, Herzog J, Kleiner Fisman G, Kubu C, Lozano A, Lyons K, et al. Deep brain stimulation: postoperative issues. *Mov Disord*. 2006; 21 Suppl 14:S219–S237. DOI: 10.1002/mds.20957.

[119] Gorgulho A, De Salles AA, Antonio AF, Frighetto L, Behnke E. Incidence of hemorrhage associated with electrophysiological studies performed using macroelectrodes and

microelectrodes in functional neurosurgery. *J Neurosurg*. 2005; 102(5):888–896. DOI: 10.3171/jns.2005.102.5.0888.

[120] Guehl D, Cuny E, Benazzouz A, Rougier A, Tison F, Machado S, et al. Side-effects of subthalamic stimulation in Parkinson's disease: clinical evolution and predictive factors. *Eur J Neurol*. 2006; 13(9):963–971. DOI: 10.1111/j.1468-1331.2006.01405.x.

[121] Falowski S, Ooi Y, Bakay RAE. Long-term evaluation of changes in operative technique and hardware-related complications with deep brain stimulation. *Neuromodulation*. 2015; 18(8):670–677. DOI: 10.1111/ner.12335.

[122] Temel Y, Ackermans L, Celik H, Spincemaille GH, van der Linden C, Walenkamp GH, et al. Management of hardware infections following deep brain stimulation. *Acta Neurochir (Wien)*. 2004; 146(4):355–361; discussion 361. DOI: 10.1007/s00701-004-0219-2.

[123] Joint C, Nandi D, Parkin S, Gregory R, Aziz T. Hardware-related problems of deep brain stimulation. *Mov Disord*. 2002; 17 Suppl 3:S175-S180. DOI: 10.1002/mds.10161.

[124] Yang Y, Jhang S, Chen C, Chen Y, Cheng C. Functional preservation of deep brain stimulation electrodes after brain shift induced by traumatic subdural haematoma - case report. *Br J Neurosurg*. 2013; 27(1):128–129. DOI: 10.3109/02688697.2012.707703.

[125] Park YS, Kim JP, Chang WS, Chang JW. Management of a DBS system in patients with traumatic brain injury: case report. *Neuromodulation*. 2011; 14(3):214–218; discussion 218. DOI: 10.1111/j.1525-1403.2011.00348.x.

[126] Benabid A, Chabardes S, Mitrofanis J, Pollak P. Deep brain stimulation of the subthalamic nucleus for the treatment of Parkinson's disease. *Lancet Neurol*. 2009; 8(1):67–81. DOI: 10.1016/S1474-4422(08)70291-6.

[127] Fraix V, Pollak P, Moro E, Chabardes S, Xie J, Ardouin C, et al. Subthalamic nucleus stimulation in tremor dominant parkinsonian patients with previous thalamic surgery. *J Neurol Neurosurg Psychiatr*. 2005; 76(2):246–248. DOI: 10.1136/jnnp.2003.022707.

[128] Krack P, Batir A, Van Blercom N, Chabardes S, Fraix V, Ardouin C, et al. Five-year follow-up of bilateral stimulation of the subthalamic nucleus in advanced Parkinson's disease. *N Engl J Med*. 2003; 349(20):1925–1934. DOI: 10.1056/NEJMoa035275.

[129] Houeto JL, Mesnage V, Mallet L, Pillon B, Gargiulo M, du Moncel ST, et al. Behavioural disorders, Parkinson's disease and subthalamic stimulation. *J Neurol Neurosurg Psychiatr*. 2002; 72(6):701–707. DOI: 10.1136/jnnp.72.6.701.

[130] Bejjani BP, Damier P, Arnulf I, Thivard L, Bonnet AM, Dormont D, et al. Transient acute depression induced by high-frequency deep-brain stimulation. *N Engl J Med*. 1999; 340(19):1476–1480. DOI: 10.1056/NEJM199905133401905.

[131] Krack P, Kumar R, Ardouin C, Dowsey PL, McVicker JM, Benabid AL, et al. Mirthful laughter induced by subthalamic nucleus stimulation. *Mov Disord*. 2001; 16(5):867–875. DOI: 10.1002/mds.1174.

[132] Herzog J, Reiff J, Krack P, Witt K, Schrader B, Müller D, et al. Manic episode with psychotic symptoms induced by subthalamic nucleus stimulation in a patient with Parkinson's disease. *Mov Disord*. 2003; 18(11):1382–1384. DOI: 10.1002/mds.10530.

[133] Romito L, Raja M, Daniele A, Contarino M, Bentivoglio A, Barbier A, et al. Transient mania with hypersexuality after surgery for high frequency stimulation of the subthalamic nucleus in Parkinson's disease. *Mov Disord*. 2002; 17(6):1371–1374. DOI: 10.1002/mds.10265.

[134] Limousin P, Krack P, Pollak P, Benazzouz A, Ardouin C, Hoffmann D, et al. Electrical stimulation of the subthalamic nucleus in advanced Parkinson's disease. *N Engl J Med*. 1998; 339(16):1105–1111. DOI: 10.1056/NEJM199810153391603.

[135] Limousin P, Pollak P, Hoffmann D, Benazzouz A, Perret JE, Benabid AL. Abnormal involuntary movements induced by subthalamic nucleus stimulation in parkinsonian patients. *Mov Disord*. 1996; 11(3):231–235. DOI: 10.1002/mds.870110303.

[136] Benabid AL, Pollak P, Gervason C, Hoffmann D, Gao DM, Hommel M, et al. Long-term suppression of tremor by chronic stimulation of the ventral intermediate thalamic nucleus. *Lancet*. 1991; 337(8738):403–406. DOI: 10.1016/0140-6736(91)91175-T.

[137] Agnesi F, Johnson M, Vitek J. Deep brain stimulation: how does it work? *Handb Clin Neurol*. 2013; 116:39–54. DOI: 10.1016/B978-0-444-53497-2.00004-8.

[138] Blahak C, Bäzner H, Capelle H, Wöhrle J, Weigel R, Hennerici M, et al. Rapid response of parkinsonian tremor to STN-DBS changes: direct modulation of oscillatory basal ganglia activity? *Mov Disord*. 2009; 24(8):1221–1225. DOI: 10.1002/mds.22536.

[139] Fasano A, Aquino C, Krauss J, Honey C, Bloem B. Axial disability and deep brain stimulation in patients with Parkinson disease. *Nat Rev Neurol*. 2015; 11(2):98–110. DOI: 10.1038/nrneurol.2014.252.

[140] Temperli P, Ghika J, Villemure J, Burkhard PR, Bogousslavsky J, Vingerhoets FJG. How do parkinsonian signs return after discontinuation of subthalamic DBS? *Neurology*. 2003; 60(1):78–81. DOI: 10.1212/WNL.60.1.78.

[141] Krauss J, Yianni J, Loher T, Aziz T. Deep brain stimulation for dystonia. *J Clin Neurophysiol*. 2004; 21(1):18–30. DOI: 10.1097/00004691-200401000-00004.

[142] Yianni J, Bain PG, Gregory RP, Nandi D, Joint C, Scott RB, et al. Post-operative progress of dystonia patients following globus pallidus internus deep brain stimulation. *Eur J Neurol*. 2003; 10(3):239–247. DOI: 10.1046/j.1468-1331.2003.00592.x.

[143] Tierney T, Abd-El-Barr MM, Stanford A, Foote K, Okun M. Deep brain stimulation and ablation for obsessive compulsive disorder: evolution of contemporary indications, targets and techniques. *Int J Neurosci*. 2014; 124(6):394–402. DOI: 10.3109/00207454.2013.852086.

[144] Servello D, Porta M, Sassi M, Brambilla A, Robertson MM. Deep brain stimulation in 18 patients with severe Gilles de la Tourette syndrome refractory to treatment: the

surgery and stimulation. *J Neurol Neurosurg Psychiatr*. 2008; 79(2):136–142. DOI: 10.1136/jnnp.2006.104067.

[145] Greenberg BD, Gabriels LA, Malone DA, Rezai AR, Friehs GM, Okun MS, et al. Deep brain stimulation of the ventral internal capsule/ventral striatum for obsessive-compulsive disorder: worldwide experience. *Mol Psychiatry*. 2010; 15(1):64–79. DOI: 10.1038/mp.2008.55.

[146] Baron M, Wichmann T, Ma D, DeLong M. Effects of transient focal inactivation of the basal ganglia in parkinsonian primates. *J Neurosci*. 2002; 22(2):592–599.

[147] Wichmann T, Bergman H, DeLong MR. The primate subthalamic nucleus. III. Changes in motor behavior and neuronal activity in the internal pallidum induced by subthalamic inactivation in the MPTP model of parkinsonism. *J Neurophysiol*. 1994; 72(2):521–530.

[148] Beurrier C, Bioulac B, Audin J, Hammond C. High-frequency stimulation produces a transient blockade of voltage-gated currents in subthalamic neurons. J *Neurophysiol*. 2001; 85(4):1351–1356.

[149] Shin DS, Samoilova M, Cotic M, Zhang L, Brotchie JM, Carlen PL. High frequency stimulation or elevated K+ depresses neuronal activity in the rat entopeduncular nucleus. *Neuroscience*. 2007; 149(1):68–86. DOI: 10.1016/j.neuroscience.2007.06.055.

[150] Dostrovsky JO, Levy R, Wu JP, Hutchison WD, Tasker RR, Lozano AM. Microstimulation-induced inhibition of neuronal firing in human globus pallidus. *J Neurophysiol*. 2000; 84(1):570–574.

[151] McIntyre C, Grill W, Sherman D, Thakor N. Cellular effects of deep brain stimulation: model-based analysis of activation and inhibition. *J Neurophysiol*. 2004; 91(4):1457–1469. DOI: 10.1152/jn.00989.2003.

[152] Histed M, Bonin V, Reid RC. Direct activation of sparse, distributed populations of cortical neurons by electrical microstimulation. *Neuron*. 2009; 63(4):508–522. DOI: 10.1016/j.neuron.2009.07.016.

[153] Sato F, Lavallée P, Lévesque M, Parent A. Single-axon tracing study of neurons of the external segment of the globus pallidus in primate. *J Comp Neurol*. 2000; 417(1):17–31. DOI: 10.1002/(SICI)1096-9861(20000131)417:1<17::AID-CNE2>3.0.CO;2-I.

[154] Anderson T, Hu B, Pittman Q, Kiss ZHT. Mechanisms of deep brain stimulation: an intracellular study in rat thalamus. *J Physiol (Lond)*. 2004; 559(1):301–313. DOI: 10.1113/jphysiol.2004.064998.

[155] Shen K, Zhu Z, Munhall A, Johnson S. Synaptic plasticity in rat subthalamic nucleus induced by high-frequency stimulation. *Synapse*. 2003; 50(4):314–319. DOI: 10.1002/syn.10274.

[156] Yamawaki N, Magill PJ, Woodhall GL, Hall SD, Stanford IM. Frequency selectivity and dopamine-dependence of plasticity at glutamatergic synapses in the subthalamic nucleus. *Neuroscience*. 2012; 203:1–11. DOI: 10.1016/j.neuroscience.2011.12.027.

[157] Creed M, Pascoli V, Lüscher C. Addiction therapy. Refining deep brain stimulation to emulate optogenetic treatment of synaptic pathology. *Science*. 2015; 347(6222):659–664. DOI: 10.1126/science.1260776.

[158] Mayberg H, Lozano A, Voon V, McNeely H, Seminowicz D, Hamani C, et al. Deep brain stimulation for treatment-resistant depression. *Neuron*. 2005; 45(5):651–660. DOI: 10.1016/j.neuron.2005.02.014.

[159] Lozano A, Mayberg H, Giacobbe P, Hamani C, Craddock RC, Kennedy S. Subcallosal cingulate gyrus deep brain stimulation for treatment-resistant depression. *Biol Psychiatry*. 2008; 64(6):461–467. DOI: 10.1016/j.biopsych.2008.05.034.

[160] Strafella A, Lozano A, Ballanger B, Poon Y, Lang A, Moro E. rCBF changes associated with PPN stimulation in a patient with Parkinson's disease: a PET study. Mov Disord. 2008; 23(7):1051–1054. DOI: 10.1002/mds.22055.

[161] Yianni J, Bradley K, Soper N, O'Sullivan V, Nandi D, Gregory R, et al. Effect of GPi DBS on functional imaging of the brain in dystonia. *J Clin Neurosci*. 2005; 12(2):137–141. DOI: 10.1016/j.jocn.2004.05.010.

[162] Kumar R, Dagher A, Hutchison WD, Lang AE, Lozano AM. Globus pallidus deep brain stimulation for generalized dystonia: clinical and PET investigation. *Neurology*. 1999; 53(4):871–874. DOI: 10.1212/WNL.53.4.871.

[163] Suetens K, Nuttin B, Gabriëls L, Van Laere K. Differences in metabolic network modulation between capsulotomy and deep-brain stimulation for refractory obsessive-compulsive disorder. *J Nucl Med*. 2014; 55(6):951–959. DOI: 10.2967/jnumed.113.126409.

[164] Rauch S, Dougherty D, Malone D, Rezai A, Friehs G, Fischman A, et al. A functional neuroimaging investigation of deep brain stimulation in patients with obsessive-compulsive disorder. *J Neurosurg*. 2006; 104(4):558–565. DOI: 10.3171/jns.2006.104.4.558.

[165] Temel Y, Visser-Vandewalle V, Kaplan S, Kozan R, Daemen MA, Blokland A, et al. Protection of nigral cell death by bilateral subthalamic nucleus stimulation. *Brain Res*. 2006; 1120(1):100–105. DOI: 10.1016/j.brainres.2006.08.082.

[166] Maesawa S, Kaneoke Y, Kajita Y, Usui N, Misawa N, Nakayama A, et al. Long-term stimulation of the subthalamic nucleus in hemiparkinsonian rats: neuroprotection of dopaminergic neurons. *J Neurosurg*. 2004; 100(4):679–687. DOI: 10.3171/jns.2004.100.4.0679.

[167] Piallat B, Benazzouz A, Benabid AL. Subthalamic nucleus lesion in rats prevents dopaminergic nigral neuron degeneration after striatal 6-OHDA injection: behavioural

and immunohistochemical studies. *Eur J Neurosci.* 1996; 8(7):1408–1414. DOI: 10.1111/j.1460-9568.1996.tb01603.x.

[168] Wallace B, Ashkan K, Heise C, Foote K, Torres N, Mitrofanis J, et al. Survival of midbrain dopaminergic cells after lesion or deep brain stimulation of the subthalamic nucleus in MPTP-treated monkeys. *Brain.* 2007; 130(8):2129–2145. DOI: 10.1093/brain/awm137.

[169] Spieles Engemann A, Steece Collier K, Behbehani M, Collier T, Wohlgenant S, Kemp C, et al. Subthalamic nucleus stimulation increases brain derived neurotrophic factor in the nigrostriatal system and primary motor cortex. *J Parkinsons Dis.* 2011; 1(1):123–136.

[170] Ho DXK, Tan Y, Tan J, Too H, Ng W. High-frequency stimulation of the globus pallidus interna nucleus modulates GFRa1 gene expression in the basal ganglia. *J Clin Neurosci.* 2014; 21(4):657–660. DOI: 10.1016/j.jocn.2013.05.024.

[171] Ashburner J, Friston KJ. Voxel-based morphometry--the methods. *Neuroimage.* 2000; 11(6):805–821. DOI: 10.1006/nimg.2000.0582.

[172] Roberts RE, Anderson E, Husain M. White matter microstructure and cognitive function. *Neuroscientist.* 2013; 19(1):8–15. DOI: 10.1177/1073858411421218.

[173] Jones D. Studying connections in the living human brain with diffusion MRI. *Cortex.* 2008; 44(8):936–952. DOI: 10.1016/j.cortex.2008.05.002.

[174] Ko J, Tang C, Eidelberg D. Brain stimulation and functional imaging with fMRI and PET. *Handb Clin Neurol.* 2013; 116:77–95. DOI: 10.1016/B978-0-444-53497-2.00008-5.

[175] Min H, Ross E, Lee K, Dennis K, Han S, Jeong J, et al. Subthalamic nucleus deep brain stimulation induces motor network BOLD activation: use of a high precision MRI guided stereotactic system for nonhuman primates. *Brain Stimul.* 2014; 7(4):603–607. DOI: 10.1016/j.brs.2014.04.007.

[176] Lin T, Carbon M, Tang C, Mogilner A, Sterio D, Beric A, et al. Metabolic correlates of subthalamic nucleus activity in Parkinson's disease. *Brain.* 2008; 131(5):1373–1380. DOI: 10.1093/brain/awn031.

[177] Friston KJ, Frith CD, Liddle PF, Frackowiak RS. Functional connectivity: the principal-component analysis of large (PET) data sets. *J Cereb Blood Flow Metab.* 1993; 13(1):5–14. DOI: 10.1038/jcbfm.1993.4.

[178] Friston K. Functional and effective connectivity: a review. *Brain Connect.* 2011; 1(1):13–36. DOI: 10.1089/brain.2011.0008.

[179] Stam CJ, Jones BF, Nolte G, Breakspear M, Scheltens P. Small-world networks and functional connectivity in Alzheimer's disease. *Cereb Cortex.* 2007; 17(1):92–99. DOI: 10.1093/cercor/bhj127.

[180] Ibrahim G, Anderson R, Akiyama T, Ochi A, Otsubo H, Singh Cadieux G, et al. Neocortical pathological high-frequency oscillations are associated with frequency-

dependent alterations in functional network topology. J *Neurophysiol*. 2013; 110(10): 2475–2483. DOI: 10.1152/jn.00034.2013.

[181] Hinkley LBN, Owen J, Fisher M, Findlay A, Vinogradov S, Nagarajan S. Cognitive impairments in schizophrenia as assessed through activation and connectivity measures of magnetoencephalography (MEG) Data. *Front Hum Neurosci*. 2010; 3:73. DOI: 10.3389/neuro.09.073.2009.

[182] Fogelson N, Li L, Li Y, Fernandez-Del-Olmo M, Santos Garcia D, Peled A. Functional connectivity abnormalities during contextual processing in schizophrenia and in Parkinson's disease. *Brain Cogn*. 2013; 82(3):243–253. DOI: 10.1016/j.bandc.2013.05.001.

[183] Sui J, Huster R, Yu Q, Segall JM, Calhoun VD. Function–structure associations of the brain: evidence from multimodal connectivity and covariance studies. *Neuroimage*. 2014; 102:11–23.

[184] Parent A, Hazrati LN. Functional anatomy of the basal ganglia. II. The place of subthalamic nucleus and external pallidum in basal ganglia circuitry. *Brain Res Brain Res Rev*. 1995; 20(1):128–154. DOI: 10.1016/0165-0173(94)00008-D.

[185] Parent A, Hazrati LN. Functional anatomy of the basal ganglia. I. The cortico-basal ganglia-thalamo-cortical loop. *Brain Res Brain Res Rev*. 1995; 20(1):91–127. DOI: 10.1016/0165-0173(94)00007-C.

[186] DeLong M, Wichmann T. Circuits and circuit disorders of the basal ganglia. *Arch Neurol*. 2007; 64(1):20–24. DOI: 10.1001/archneur.64.1.20.

[187] Jech R, Urgosík D, Tintera J, Nebuzelský A, Krásenský J, Liscák R, et al. Functional magnetic resonance imaging during deep brain stimulation: a pilot study in four patients with Parkinson's disease. *Mov Disord*. 2001; 16(6):1126–1132. DOI: 10.1002/mds.1217.

[188] Stefurak T, Mikulis D, Mayberg H, Lang A, Hevenor S, Pahapill P, et al. Deep brain stimulation for Parkinson's disease dissociates mood and motor circuits: a functional MRI case study. *Mov Disord*. 2003; 18(12):1508–1516. DOI: 10.1002/mds.10593.

[189] Phillips M, Baker K, Lowe M, Tkach J, Cooper S, Kopell B, et al. Parkinson disease: pattern of functional MR imaging activation during deep brain stimulation of subthalamic nucleus--initial experience. *Radiology*. 2006; 239(1):209–216. DOI: 10.1148/radiol.2391041990.

[190] Kahan J, Mancini L, Urner M, Friston K, Hariz M, Holl E, et al. Therapeutic subthalamic nucleus deep brain stimulation reverses cortico-thalamic coupling during voluntary movements in Parkinson's disease. *PLoS One*. 2012; 7(12):e50270. DOI: 10.1371/journal.pone.0050270.

[191] Paschali A, Constantoyannis C, Angelatou F, Vassilakos P. Perfusion brain SPECT in assessing motor improvement after deep brain stimulation in Parkinson's disease. *Acta Neurochir (Wien)*. 2013; 155(3):497–505. DOI: 10.1007/s00701-012-1610-z.

[192] Ma Y, Tang C, Spetsieris P, Dhawan V, Eidelberg D. Abnormal metabolic network activity in Parkinson's disease: test-retest reproducibility. *J Cereb Blood Flow Metab*. 2007; 27(3):597–605. DOI: 10.1038/sj.jcbfm.9600358.

[193] Wu P, Wang J, Peng S, Ma Y, Zhang H, Guan Y, et al. Metabolic brain network in the Chinese patients with Parkinson's disease based on 18F-FDG PET imaging. *Parkinsonism Relat Disord*. 2013; 19(6):622–627. DOI: 10.1016/j.parkreldis.2013.02.013.

[194] Hashimoto T, Elder C, Okun M, Patrick S, Vitek J. Stimulation of the subthalamic nucleus changes the firing pattern of pallidal neurons. *J Neurosci*. 2003; 23(5):1916–1923.

[195] Li S, Arbuthnott GW, Jutras MJ, Goldberg JA, Jaeger D. Resonant antidromic cortical circuit activation as a consequence of high-frequency subthalamic deep-brain stimulation. *J Neurophysiol*. 2007; 98(6):3525–3537. DOI: 10.1152/jn.00808.2007.

[196] Stefani A, Fedele E, Galati S, Pepicelli O, Frasca S, Pierantozzi M, et al. Subthalamic stimulation activates internal pallidus: evidence from cGMP microdialysis in PD patients. *Ann Neurol*. 2005; 57(3):448–452. DOI: 10.1002/ana.20402.

[197] Stefani A, Fedele E, Galati S, Raiteri M, Pepicelli O, Brusa L, et al. Deep brain stimulation in Parkinson's disease patients: biochemical evidence. *J Neural Transm Suppl*. 2006; (70): 401–408.

[198] Stefani A, Fedele E, Pierantozzi M, Galati S, Marzetti F, Peppe A, et al. Reduced GABA content in the motor thalamus during effective deep brain stimulation of the subthalamic nucleus. *Front Syst Neurosci*. 2011; 5:17. DOI: 10.3389/fnsys.2011.00017.

[199] Galati S, Mazzone P, Fedele E, Pisani A, Peppe A, Pierantozzi M, et al. Biochemical and electrophysiological changes of substantia nigra pars reticulata driven by subthalamic stimulation in patients with Parkinson's disease. *Eur J Neurosci*. 2006; 23(11):2923–2928. DOI: 10.1111/j.1460-9568.2006.04816.x.

[200] Fedele E, Raiteri M. In vivo studies of the cerebral glutamate receptor/NO/cGMP pathway. *Prog Neurobiol*. 1999; 58(1):89–120. DOI: 10.1016/S0301-0082(98)00077-X.

[201] Montgomery E. Effects of GPi stimulation on human thalamic neuronal activity. Clin Neurophysiol. 2006; 117(12):2691–2702. DOI: 10.1016/j.clinph.2006.08.011.

Chapter 3

ONS and DBS for the Treatment of Chronic Cluster Headache

Giuseppe Messina, Angelo Franzini,
Alberto Proietti Cecchini and Massimo Leone

Additional information is available at the end of the chapter

http://dx.doi.org/10.5772/64482

Abstract

Research focus: Chronic cluster headache (CCH) is a pathological entity leading to a severe degree of disability. It is characterized by pain attacks occurring daily or spaced out by remission periods of <1 month, contrarily to the episodic form. When the condition results to be refractory to conservative treatments (both prophylactic and abortive treatments) and when such condition is present for at least 2 years, surgical treatment is suggested.

Research methods: We here report our institutional experience with regard to both occipital nerve stimulation (ONS) and deep brain stimulation (DBS) for the treatment of the disease.

Results/findings of the research: 15 out of 28 (65%) patients submitted to ONS had ≥50% reduction in 32 headache number per day and were considered responders; 12 out of 17 patients (70%) submitted to phyp DBS showed long-last improvement.

Main conclusions and recommendations: Although no valid predictive factor is available at the moment, due to the lack of prospective and randomized studies, both procedures seem to constitute safe and valid treatments for such disabling condition.

Keywords: cluster headache, occipital nerve stimulation, deep brain stimulation, hypothalamus

1. Introduction

Cluster headache (CH) is characterized by severe strictly unilateral headaches lasting 15–180 minutes, and accompanied by autonomic signs (rhinorrhea, lacrimation, and conjunctival injection). CH appears most commonly in its episodic form (pain bouts occurring from once every day to eight times a day, with pain periods lasting about 1–2 months). The chronic form of CH (CCH) is instead characterized by pain attacks which recur over >1 year without remission periods or with remission periods lasting <1 month [1]. Some patients affected from the chronic form become drug-resistant, with subsequent severe disability in activity of daily life. In the past, different ablative surgical procedures have been employed, but with overall poor results due to the high incidence of adverse events [2]. For more than a decade, deep brain stimulation of the posterior hypothalamic region (pHyp) has been employed to treat such patients at several centers, with encouraging results [3]. In the past years, however, a less invasive procedure, occipital nerve stimulation (ONS), has been effective as well [4–7]. Such procedure is now currently proposed as first-line surgical treatment, before the employment of deep brain stimulation (DBS). At present, no prospective randomized controlled trial is available for either procedure, although one such study is ongoing at present with regard to ONS [8]. It is thus not possible at the moment to draw any certain conclusion about the predictive factors which could influence the outcome in both procedures, but results available to date are encouraging. Correct selection criteria, however, appear of utmost importance to maximize results.

1.1. Occipital nerve stimulation

The rationale for the employment of electrical current applied to the great occipital nerve to treat headache relies on the evidence of convergence of trigeminal and cervical afferents on second-order neurons located on the so-called trigeminocervical complex (neural columns extending from the trigeminal nucleus caudalis to the C2 spinal segment) [9]; furthermore, steroids injected into the suboccipital region were able to improve some types of headaches, including CH [10]. Several reports suggest that ONS is an effective procedure for drug-resistant chronic CH patients [4–7]. We began to use this surgical procedure in 2004 at our Institution, proposing it before the more invasive DBS.

2. Materials and methods

Inclusion criteria for ONS at our Institution were drug-resistant CCH, that is daily or almost daily attacks in the past year and resistance to all known prophylactic drugs for such condition, including verapamil, lithium carbonate, methysergide, valproate, topiramate, gabapentin, melatonin, pizotifen, indomethacin, and others including sphenopalatine ganglion blockade [11, 12]. Long-term steroid cycles were also used in all patients at the expense of development of well-known related side effects (arterial hypertension, peptic ulcers, bone fractures, weight increase, insomnia, psychosis, glaucoma, and skin eruptions). Although we think successful

http://dx.doi.org/10.5772/64482

occipital nerve blockade was one of the factors which initially encouraged the use of the procedure in CH, it was not used as a selection criterion at our center (and the same applies to external ONS trial) due to the uncertainty with regard to its predictive positive effect.

Twenty-eight patients satisfied the criteria underwent ONS system implantation at our Institute from March 2004 to February 2013. They included 23 men and 5 women. The mean age at operation was 43 years, the mean duration of chronic CH was 6.6 years (range: 1–27), and the mean number of attacks per day was 5.4 (range: 2–10) (**Table 1**). All patients had normal neurological examination and normal cerebral MRI; psychiatric and psychological evaluations were negative in all cases. The five women included were not pregnant. All patients gave written informed consent to the procedure.

Pt. No	AGE	GENDER	DURATION OF CHRONIC CH (years)	No OF ATTACKS PER DAY	FOLLOW UP	RESPONDERS (Y/ N)	IMPROVEMENT (%)	TIME TO IMPROVEMENT (weeks)	MEDTRONIK=M; SAINT JUDE=SJ	BILATERAL STIMULATION	STEROIDS AFTER ONS	EMPTY BATTERY	ADVERSE EVENTS
1	56	M	4	4	NA	NA	NA	NA	M	N	NA	NA	-
2	69	M	4	2	NA	NA	NA	NA	M	N	NA	NA	-
3	24	M	1	4	NA	NA	NA	NA	M	N	NA	NA	-
4	27	M	3	6	NA	NA	NA	NA	M	N	NA	NA	-
5	45	F	5	5	NA	NA	NA	NA	M	N	NA	NA	-
6	56	M	3	5	8,6	N	NO	-	M	N	Y	N*	-
7	44	M	9	4	8,0	Y	EPISODIC CH	12	M	Y	N	Yes (1)	electrode migration
8	53	M	18	3	9,4	Y	SPORADIC HEADACHES	14	M	Y	N	Yes (1)	-
9	53	M	3	4	7,8	Y	SPORADIC HEADACHES	18	M	Y	N	Yes (1)	wire decubitus
10	37	F	5	6	8,3	Y	EPISODIC CH	9	M	Y	N	Yes (2)	-
11	43	M	5	6	8,1	N	NO	-	M	Y	Y	Yes (1)	electrode migration
12	33	M	7	3	10,3	N	NO	-	M	N	Y	Yes (2)	-
13	33	M	10	4	7,1	Y	SPORADIC HEADACHES	32	M	Y	N	Yes (1)	-
14	31	M	11	3	7,0	Y	SPORADIC HEADACHES	12	M→SJ	Y	N	Yes (2)	electrode migration
15	53	M	11	7	6,9	N	NO	-	M	Y	Y	N*	-
16	48	M	3	8	6,6	Y	SPORADIC HEADACHES	2	M→SJ	Y	Y	Yes (2)	wire decubitus
17	38	M	2	8	6,5	N	NO	-	M	Y	Y	Yes (1)	-
18	33	F	3	8	6,4	Y	SPORADIC HEADACHES	9	M	Y	N	Yes (2)	-
19	35	M	4	4	6,1	N	NO	-	M	Y	Y	Yes (1)	
20	33	M	4	10	5,7	N	NO	-	M	Y	N	N	electrode migration
21	49	M	10	6	5,5	Y	SPORADIC HEADACHES	8	M	Y	N	N	-
22	54	M	27	6	4,5	Y	SPORADIC HEADACHES	1	M	Y	N	N	-
23	30	M	4	7	5,1	Y	EPISODIC CH	37	M	Y	N	Yes (1)	electrode migration
24	53	M	2	7	5,1	Y	SPORADIC HEADACHES	3	M	N	N	N	-
25	29	M	10	8	4,5	N	NO	-	M	Y	Y	N	electrode migration
26	44	M	10	4	3,0	Y	SPORADIC HEADACHES	9	SJ	N	N	Yes (2)	-
27	53	M	5	6	3,0	Y	SPORADIC HEADACHES	21	SJ	Y	N	Yes (2)	electrode *plus* wire malfunctioning
28	50	M	3	3	2,8	Y	60	3	SJ	Y	N	Yes (1)	-
	43		6,6	5,4	5,2			6.7					

Table 1. Clinical and outcome features in ONS patients

The first five implanted patients received ONS for less than 6 months with poor results, so we decided to offer them hypothalamic stimulation; at that time, it was shown that in neurovascular headaches ONS was only effective at short-term follow-up [13]. These five patients are not considered in the analysis.

3. Surgery

The ONS surgical procedure varies from center to center. We here describe the procedure employed at our Institution, taking into account the validity and safety of other methodologies. Ours has also been described in a previous report [14]. The patient is placed in a prone position, and the Mayfield head holder system is used to fix the head. Bony prominences must be padded to prevent postoperative lesions of nondependent skin and nerves. The head is positioned in line with the neck and posterior thoracic region and chest to avoid skin creases and curvatures, which could be cumbersome and lengthen the procedure. The Mayfield head holder is positioned in the parietal region bilaterally so as not to interfere with the leads' positioning. We always perform bilateral ONS to anticipate eventual side shift of symptomatology. Quadripolar bilateral electrodes or one longer octopolar electrode is employed. A vertical skin incision is made in the posterior cervical region in the midline from 1 cm above to 1 cm below the external occipital protuberance (EOP). The greater occipital nerve (GON) is usually present about 4 cm lateral to the midline turning in a slight mediolateral direction before dividing into a medial and a lateral branch about 1 cm above the EOP (**Figure 1**). Two symmetric vertical incisions are then made 7 cm lateral to the EOP bilaterally. The cervical fascia located superficial to the trapezius and splenius capitis muscles is exposed after blunt dissection of subcutaneous tissue in the region.

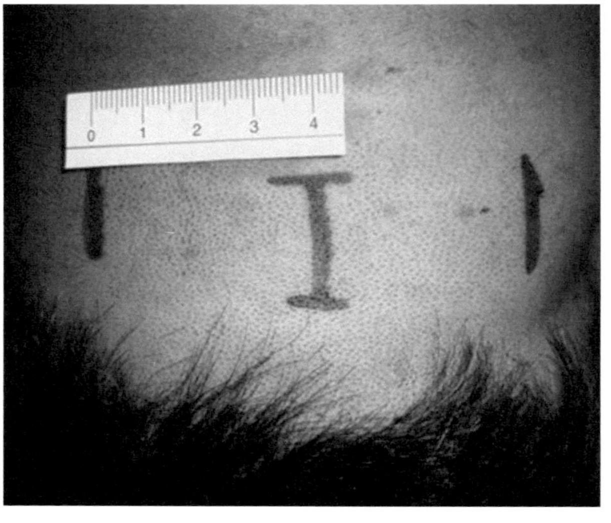

Figure 1. Preoperative GON localization.

A Tuohy needle is then inserted from each lateral incision to the midline incision, allowing the insertion of the electrode after the removal of the stylet. The wires connected to the electrodes are then tunneled together in a caudal direction along the occipital and neck midline until about the middle dorsal level.

We do not use anchorage devices but in the cervical region we fix both electrodes to the underlying fascia with nonresorbable stitches to prevent their caudal dislodgement; and relief loops are made at both this site and at more subcutaneous caudal sites during tunneling passages to prevent excessive discomfort to the patient, and possible leads' fracture. For the same purpose (avoid excessive strain on the system), we use 95 cm length connection wires. We create a little subcutaneous pocket at the level of the connectors (whenever present) between main leads and connection cables to avoid possible skin erosions underlying them. Another incision is made in the midline at the lumbar level and, at this point, the two connection cables diverge on each side to the site of the subcutaneous pockets where internal pulse generators (IPGs) will be located.

One or two IPGs (Soletra, Medtronic, Libra, St Jude, Activa PC, Medtronic, Libra xp, St Jude) can be used. Of course, we leave the connection cables and the IPGs in site, when it becomes necessary to convert ONS into hypothalamic deep brain stimulation. Subcutaneous pockets for IPGs are made approximately 4 cm above the iliac crest at the level of the external oblique muscle, paying attention not to jeopardize the latter muscle and not to cause excessive bleeding and postoperative pain.

In the postoperative period, all patients underwent plain cranial radiographies to verify the adequate leads' positioning, and IPGs were switched on, progressively increasing voltage or current intensity until adequate paresthesia coverage was reached in the somatic GON territory.

4. Results

Following implant, we turned on IPGs after a median of 3.3 days (range: 0–14 days) because of the lack of attacks in such postoperative period. Stimulation was started once attacks reappeared and improvement occurred after a median of 6.7 weeks (range: 1–37 weeks; **Table 1**).

All patients perceived paresthesias in somatic areas innervated by the occipital nerve. Stimulation parameters were set according to the patient's tolerability. When induced perceived paresthesia became unbearable for the patient at some time after activation the amplitude was reduced accordingly. No specific stimulation pattern was found to be predictive of long-term efficacy; in fact, many stimulation adjustments were necessary to achieve optimal results.

After a median follow-up of 5.2 years (range: 2.8–10), 15 (65%) patients had ≥50% reduction in headache number per day (responders). Eleven (47%) responders have a stable condition with only sporadic attacks; in three other patients, chronic CH turned into episodic CH; the remaining responder had a 60% reduction in headache number per day (**Table 1**).

Eight (34.7%) patients were nonresponders. Five of these showed a ≥50% reduction in headache number per day in the first months after implant: in four patients the initial improvement lasted up to 12 months after ONS; in the remaining patient such improvement lasted 48 months.

After ONS 15 (65%) patients stopped steroidal treatment while the remaining eight received short-term steroid courses. All patients needed to maintain prophylactic treatment for CH.

5. Discussion

As stated above, at long follow-up examinations, our results show that ONS is able to produce long-lasting improvement in a large number of patients (65%); more importantly, in 47% of patients a stable condition with sporadic attacks is reported.

It is well known that a placebo effect cannot be excluded in CH patients [15], and it is not possible to rule out that the improvement observed is part of the natural course of the disease; furthermore, for long-term observational purposes, blinding in such cases is not possible because paresthesias are necessary to achieve positive results. Anyway, two elements point to a real effectiveness of ONS: the long-term follow-up of the present series (and of other series reported in literature) and the relapse of symptoms at battery's exhaustion.

Several studies report different long-term outcomes. In the study of Magis et al. [5] of 2011, responders' rate was as high as 78.6% (11 of 14 patients) after a mean follow-up of 36.8 months. The same author recently published a very long term follow-up extension of such study including 10 patients [7]; of these, four (40%) evolved to an episodic form and six (60%) remained chronic but with a reduction of about 70%. Fontaine et al. [6] reported a responders' rate of 76.9% (11 of 13 patients) after a mean follow-up of 14.6 months and Muller et al. [4] reported a responders' rate of 90% (9 of 10 patients) after a mean follow-up of 12 months. A lower percentage of responders, 35.7% (5 of 14 patients), after a median follow-up of 17. 5 months has been reported in another study [16]. Such differences in outcome could most probably reflect differences in follow-up lengths (given the substantial standardization of the procedure). Note that in our study five patients became resistant after several months of improvement; one patient became resistant to ONS after a 4-year improvement. Our experience thus witnesses the possibility of developing tolerance to ONS, but unfortunately we did not find any significant factor which could be considered a reliable predictor of tolerance or unresponsiveness.

All the patients considered responders in our series could stop steroid therapy and only one third of them needed steroids for short periods. It is worth noticing that the daily Sumatriptan injection consumption was markedly reduced after ONS. It is well known that the prolonged use of these drugs can lead to life-threatening side effects, and in fact this is actually considered among selection criteria for ONS in drug-resistant chronic CH patients.

Empty batteries were the most common AE (adverse event) (and it is in the existent literature). This is due to the high voltage or current intensity necessary to obtain satisfactory results; anyway, in long-term responders, we have begun to implant rechargeable IPGs in such patients.

The exact mechanisms underlying the beneficial effects of ONS in drCCH patients are still under investigation; the co-presence of trigeminal and cervical somatic input to second-order neurons located in the so-called trigeminocervical complex, extending from the trigeminal nucleus caudalis to the C2 cervical nuclear complex, could explain the role of modulating the myelomere C2 in the beneficial effect of ONS [17]; Magis et al. [18] in 2011 investigated the FDG-PET modifications in 10 patients submitted to ONS after a minimum of 6-month follow-up. In CCH patients at baseline (compared to healthy subjects), hypermetabolism was noticed in the ipsilateral hypothalamus, midbrain, and ipsilateral lower pons. In all patients, this picture normalized after ONS, and the hypothalamus was the only exception. It was also noticed that the metabolism of perigenual anterior cingulate cortex (PACC) was hyperactive in ONS responders compared to nonresponders. The authors thus hypothesized the pure symptomatic role of ONS in CCH patients (given the lack of changes in the hypothalamus), a slow neuromodulatory role of ONS on the "pain neuromatrix" (also involving the pACC), and, as such, a specific analgesic effect acting at central dysfunctional pain control centers.

6. pHyp DBS

Two main original observations initially led to the identification of the posterior hypothalamus as having a pivotal role in the genesis of cluster headache: its activation, as revealed in brain PET studies, during CH attacks [19], and the evidence of an increased neuronal density at this site measured with voxel-based MRI morphometry [20]. Furthermore, CH attacks often recur following a certain circadian rhythm and cluster periods occur circannually. So, it was initially hypothesized that hypothalamic "biologic clocks" may be involved in the pathogenesis of CH [21]. The aim of the stereotactic procedure (pHyp DBS) performed at our Institute was thus to inhibit the posterior hypothalamic neuronal pools, thought to be responsible (when hyperactive) for the disease. Several institutional experiences have been reported since our initial observations, and overall results are encouraging. To date, pHyp DBS is offered to patients not responding to ONS, since the first obviously constitutes a more risky and invasive surgical procedure.

7. Materials and methods

Selection criteria for pHyp DBS are quite uniform among all centers employing such technique; at our Institution, we use the following criteria: (1) the presence of diagnostic criteria for CCH according to the International Headache Society [1]; (2) inadequate relief from prophylactic therapy, including verapamil, lithium, sodium valproate, methysergide, topiramate, gabapentin, nonsteroidal anti-inflammatory drugs such as indomethacin, and corticosteroids; (3) CCH lasting at least 2 years; (4) unsatisfactory relief from abortive therapy, including oxygen, Sumatriptan, and opioids; and (5) failure of occipital nerve stimulation therapy for at least 1 year.

At our Institution, 19 patients satisfying such criteria (15 men; mean age at surgery: 42 years; mean duration of CCH: 3 years) underwent pHyp DBS. Psychiatric and neuropsychological examinations were normal in all of them. All patients gave written informed consent for the procedure.

8. Surgery

Brain MRI images, obtained preoperatively, were transferred to the operating room workstation (StealthStation; Medtronic Sofamor Danek, Memphis, TN). After positioning of the stereotactic frame around the patient's head, computed tomographic (CT) scans were taken. MRI and CT images were then merged using the Framelink 4.0 software (Medtronic). From the resulting three-dimensional reconstruction, the exact position of the anterior commissure-posterior commissure line and the coordinates of the target were derived. pHyp region's coordinates were 3 mm behind the midcommissural point (Y), 5 mm below the midcommissural point (Z) , and 2 mm lateral to the midline. A 7 mm hand-driven burr hole is then made at 3 cm lateral to the scalp midline and about 2 cm anterior to the coronal suture; after coagulation of the dura mater a rigid cannula is inserted to within 10 mm of the target; the quadripolar electrode was then inserted to the target. We usually perform intraoperative stimulation (beginning at 60 μs, 180 Hz, up to 7 V) to verify tolerability and side effects. Amplitudes above 4 V usually produced ipsilateral eye version with consequent diplopia. Throughout the procedure, pupils, heart rate, blood pressure, electroencephalogram, body temperature, and respiratory function were monitored. Cerebral CT was performed immediately after implant; MRI was performed within 48 hours after surgery and merged with postoperative CT scan to accurately verify the position of electrode's contacts (**Figures 2** and **3**). Postoperatively, patients were left without active stimulation till insurgence of CH attacks; they were not provided prophylactic medication in the meantime.

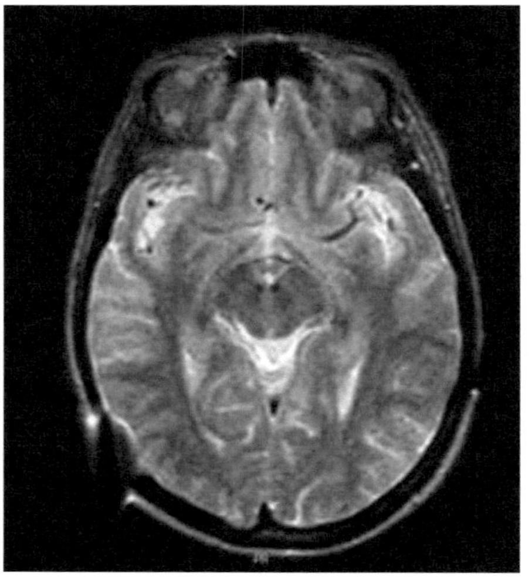

Figure 2. Postoperative MRI showing bilateral pHyp electrodes' tips localization in a CCH patient.

Hospitalization lasted about 10–20 days in order to allow for monitoring of CH attacks, blood pressure, heart rate and function, temperature, sleep-wake cycle, body weight, electrolyte balance, and hormone levels. These variables were checked at regular intervals after discharge.

Patients also kept a diary reporting headache attacks, drug use, and adverse events. Parameters' settings (in particular amplitude and current intensity) were then programmed taking into account the minimum level providing efficacy or the maximum level tolerated.

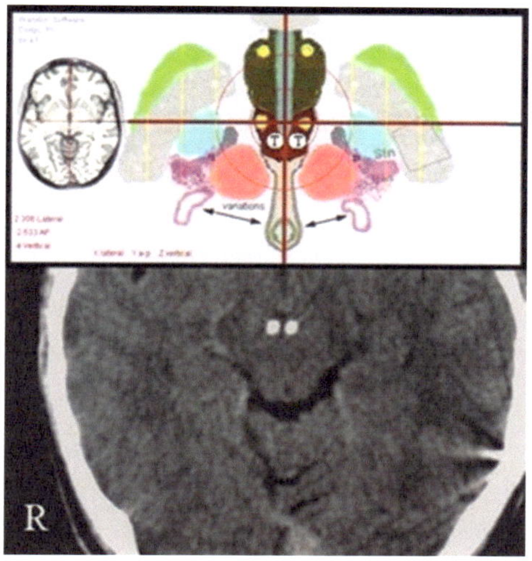

Figure 3. Upper: our institutional localization system applied to posterior hypothalamic region. Lower: Postoperative MRI-CT merged image showing the localization of bilateral posterior hypothalamic electrodes.

9. Results

Outcomes relating to our series and related details can be more systematically found by Leone [21] (**Table 2**). Briefly, the median follow-up was 8.7 years; one of our patients died of septic shock caused by Legionella infection. He was, however, free of CH bouts. Due to the infection, the entire DBS system was removed from another patient. In the remaining 17 patients, 6 (35%) subsequently had fewer than one attack every 3 months; in 5 of them, the IPG had been off (unactivated) for a median of 3 years, after a median of 6.4 years of active stimulation with continuous improvement. Another 6 patients (35%) did not experience daily attacks, instead suffering from attacks lasting from 2 to 5 months, followed by remission lasting from 5 to 10 months.

Five of 17 patients (30%) were not responders despite experiencing daily CH attacks after an initial improvement period. After DBS implantation, patients remained unstimulated for a median of two days (range: 0–12 days), given the lack of pain bouts in this period. Stimulation was initiated once pain attacks reappeared; improvement occurred 2–16 weeks later. As for ONS, several parameter adjustments were necessary to optimize clinical results.

Patient no./ side	Age at operation (y)	Sex	Chronic for (y) a	Follow-up (y)	Headache response: current and (headache status in 2006)	Current stimulation status	Time to response after stimulator on (d)	Prophylaxis	Amplitude (V)	Adverse events
1 L	39	M	4	12	Recurrence in periods (painfree)	off	30	Verapamil		
1 R	40			11	Recurrence in periods (painfree)	on	1		1.6	Right: electrode displaced; electrode replaced. Pulse generator infection; replaced
2 L	50	M	4	11	Almost painfree (pain-free)	off	72	Methysergide		
3 L	63	F	7	11	Almost painfree (pain-free)	Off	32	Verapamil		
4 R	52	M	5	10	Recurrence in periods (1 attack every 2 d)	on	42	Methysergide plus Verapamil	2.6	Electrode mal-positioned; repositioned
5 L	30	M	2	10	Almost painfree (pain-free)	off	22	None		
6 L	45	M	2	NA	NA (pain-free	NA	43	None		
7 L	27	F	1	9	Tolerance on both sides (sporadic attacks)	OFF	38	Verapamil		Reduced right arm strength. Electrode (right) displacement after trauma; infection after electrode replacement. One seizure 24 h after replacement
7 R				9			32			
8 R	25	M	1	9	Almost painfree (pain-free)	OFF	44	None		
9 R	47	M	3	8	Recurrence in periods	ON	23	Lithium	2.0	

http://dx.doi.org/10.5772/64482

					(painfree)					
10 L	43	M	10	8	Almost painfree (1 mild attack per day)	ON	56	Verapamil	2.6	Subtle transient asymptomatic hemorrhage in third ventricle
11 R	49	M	1	8	Recurrence in periods (sporadic attacks)	ON	37	Verapamil	2.6	
12 L	36	M	3	8	Recurrence in periods (painfree)	ON	62	Topiramate plus lamotrigine	4.5	
13 L	24	M	1	8	Tolerance on both sides (Sporadic attacks)	OFF	40	Verapamil		
13 R	26			7						
14 R	50	M	1	8	Tolerance (painfree)	ON	48	Lamotrigine plus prednisolone	4.6	
15 R	57	M	4	8	Almost painfree (pain-free)	OFF	86	None		
16 L	70	M	4	7	No (improvement (1 attack per day)	OFF	b	Ergotamine		
17	39	F	2	NA	NA	removed	NA	None	NA	Electrode infection and transient hemiparesis; electrode removed
18 L	28	M	3	6	30–40% reduction in headache frequency and intensity on both sides	on	95	Verapamil plus amitriptyline	1.0	
18 R						on			3.5	Electrode infection (right) and transient hemiparesis
19 L	45	F	5	6	Recurrenc	on	72	Verapamil	2.7	

					e in periods					
Mea n	42		3	8.7			47		2.8	

Table 2. Clinical and outcome fatures in DBS patients.

10. Discussion

Our experience has shown that hypothalamic stimulation produces long-lasting improvement in a high proportion of patients (70%). Stimulation seems to be tolerated for years after implantation. It is worth noticing that in some patients, after several years of stimulation, a persistent, almost pain-free, condition could be maintained in off stimulation conditions. Bilateral chronic CH seems to predict poor response to hypothalamic stimulation. After a median of almost 9 years (range: 6–12 years), 70% of our patients were improved: six patients (35%) were in a persistent almost pain-free state, and in six patients (35%), CCH condition turned into episodic CH. In most patients, prophylactic drugs were required to maintain improvement, whereas they were ineffective before surgery. High-dose steroids led to some relief, although accompanied by adverse effects. The 12 improved patients discontinued steroid therapy. When the stimulator was switched off (condition blinded to the patient), the crises returned and the same thing occurred when the stimulator batteries ran down. After IPGs replacement, these patients improved again. Worsening of attacks also occurred after electrode displacement in two patients. Taking into account these findings, a placebo effect seems unlikely. So far, over 50 chronic drug-resistant CH patients are documented to have received hypothalamic stimulation; marked improvements have occurred in 50–100% of cases (with a median follow-up of 15.8 months) (range: 12–33 months) [22–25].

It is noteworthy that in five of six of our persistently almost pain-free patients, this state is now maintained even though the stimulator has been off for several years. It should thus be proposed that after a long period of stimulation (median 6.4 years), in long-term responsive patients turning off stimulation should be tried. In five cases, headache frequency did not worsen. Such patients could tolerate a low-frequency attack (which was much better than the previous situation of intractable attacks several times daily), which also responded promptly to Sumatriptan injection.

This was not the case in the early years after implantation, when in all cases attacks reappeared when the stimulator was turned off. In six patients, the condition reverted to episodic CH but the patient needed to continue stimulation. The outcomes in these two subgroups suggest that years of continuous hypothalamic stimulation can change the course of the illness. Five of our patients (30%) were not responders. Patients without response to hypothalamic stimulation have been reported by other authors [22–25], but no reliable predictive factor is available so far. Four (80%) of our unsuccessful cases had bilateral CH, and three developed tolerance to hypothalamic stimulation after 1–2 years of improvement.

These observations suggest that bilateral CH predicts poor response to hypothalamic stimulation. As far as coordinates are concerned, Seijo et al. [26] modified them to avoid the lateral ventricle wall, also extending the stimulated brain area to the lateral hypothalamus implicated in pain modulation. The good results in this small series are encouraging, but longer follow-up is required. Our experience is that small changes in contacts and electrode position do not have influence on therapeutic response.

11. Conclusions

ONS and pHyp DBS should be proposed to drug-refractory CCH patients according to the above-mentioned criteria; a randomized trial is actually ongoing to determine the effectiveness of ONS in such patients [8], but, to date, no prospective and randomized trial is available for both procedures to determine eventual positive or negative predictive factors in the outcome of the disease; thus, our observations could be still considered useful until new findings will come.

The role of a pure symptomatic role of ONS seems to be a likely observation, whereas long-term effectiveness of pHyp DBS, especially considering patients with positive results despite off-stimulation condition, suggests a possible role in plastic neuronal changes induced by such procedure. Prospective and randomized studies are, of course, necessary, to date, to clarify the issue of nonresponder patients, thus refining the selection criteria and improving outcome in more carefully selected drug-resistant CCH patients.

Author details

Giuseppe Messina[1*], Angelo Franzini[1], Alberto Proietti Cecchini[2] and Massimo Leone[2]

*Address all correspondence to: giusmex@gmail.com

1 Department of Neurosurgery, Fondazione IRCCS Istituto Neurologico Carlo Besta, Milan, Italy

2 Department of Neurology, Fondazione IRCCS Istituto Neurologico Carlo Besta, Milan, Italy

References

[1] Headache Classification Committee of the International Headache Society. The International Classification of Headache Disorders, 2nd ed. Cephalalgia 2004; 24 (Supplement 1): 1–160.

[2] O'Brien M, Kirpatrick PJ, MacCabe JJ. Trigeminal nerve section for chronic migraine neuralgia. In: Cluster Headache and Related Conditions. Olesen J, Goadsby PJ (Eds.) Oxford University Press, Oxford, UK, 1999; 291–295.

[3] Franzini A, Messina G, Cordella R, Marras C, Broggi G. Deep brain stimulation of the posteromedial hypothalamus: indications, long-term results, and neurophysiological considerations. Neurosurg Focus 2010; 29(2): E13.

[4] Mueller OM, Gaul C, Katsarava Z, Diener HC, Sure U, Gasser T. Occipital nerve stimulation for the treatment of chronic cluster headache—lessons learned from 18 months experience. Cent Eur Neurosurg 2011; 72(2): 84–89.

[5] Magis D, Gerardy PY, Remacle JM, Schoenen J. Sustained effectiveness of occipital nerve stimulation in drug-resistant chronic cluster headache. Headache 2011; 51(8): 1191–1201.

[6] Fontaine D, Christophe Sol J, Raoul S, Fabre N, Geraud G, Magne C, Sakarovitch C, Lanteri-Minet M. Treatment of refractory chronic cluster headache by chronic occipital nerve stimulation. Cephalalgia 2011; 31(10): 1101–1105.

[7] Magis D, Gérard P, Schoenen J. Invasive occipital nerve stimulation for refractory chronic cluster headache: what evolution at long-term? Strengths and weaknesses of the method. J Headache Pain 2016; 17(1): 8.

[8] Wilbrink LA, Teernstra OP, Haan J, van Zwet EW, Evers SM, Spincemaille GH, Veltink PH, Mulleners W, Brand R, Huygen FJ, Jensen RH, Paemeleire K, Goadsby PJ, Visser-Vandewalle V, Ferrari MD. Occipital nerve stimulation in medically intractable, chronic cluster headache. The ICON study: rationale and protocol of a randomised trial. . Cephalalgia 2013; 33(15): 1238–1247.

[9] Piovesan EJ, Kowacs PA, Oshinsky ML. Convergence of cervical and trigeminal sensory afferents. Curr Pain Headache Rep 2003; 7(5): 377–383.

[10] Ambrosini A, Vandenheede M, Rossi P, Aloj F, Sauli E, Pierelli F, Schoenen J. Suboccipital injection with a mixture of rapid- and long-acting steroids in cluster headache: a double-blind placebo-controlled study. Pain 2005; 118(1–2): 92–96.

[11] Leone M, May A, Franzini A, Broggi G, Dodick D, Rapoport A, Goadsby PJ, Schoenen J, Bonavita V, Bussone G. Deep brain stimulation for intractable chronic cluster headache: proposals for patient selection. Cephalalgia 2004; 24 (11): 934–937.

[12] May A, Leone M, Áfra J, Frese A, Linde M, Sándor PS, Evers S, Goadsby PJ. EFNS guideline on the treatment of cluster headache and other trigemino-autonomic cephalgias. Eur J Neurol 2006; 13: 1066–1077.

[13] Matharu MS, Bartsch T, Ward N, Frackowiak RS, Weiner R, Goadsby PJ. Central neuromodulation in chronic migraine patients with suboccipital stimulators: a PET study. Brain 2004; 127(Pt 1): 220–230.

[14] Franzini A, Messina G, Leone M, Broggi G. Occipital nerve stimulation (ONS). Surgical technique and prevention of late electrode migration. Acta Neurochir (Wien) 2009; 151(7): 861–865.

[15] Law S, Derry S, Moore RA. Triptans for acute cluster headache. Cochrane Database Syst Rev 2014; (4): CD008042.

[16] Burns B, Watkins L, Goadsby PJ. Treatment of intractable chronic cluster headache by occipital nerve stimulation in 14 patients. Neurology 2009; 72(4): 341–345.

[17] Le Doare K, Akerman S, Holland PR, Lasalandra MP, Bergerot A, Classey JD, Knight YE, Goadsby PJ. Occipital afferent activation of second order neurons in the trigeminocervical complex in rat. Neurosci Lett 2006, 403: 73–77.

[18] Magis D, Bruno MA, Fumal A, Gérardy PY, Hustinx R, Laureys S, Schoenen J. Central modulation in cluster headache patients treated with occipital nerve stimulation: an FDG-PET study. BMC Neurol 2011; 11: 25.

[19] May A, Bahra A, Büchel C, Frackowiak RS, Goadsby PJ. Hypothalamic activation in cluster headache attacks. Lancet 1998; 352(9124): 275–278.

[20] May A, Ashburner J, Büchel C, McGonigle DJ, Friston KJ, Frackowiak RS, Goadsby PJ. Correlation between structural and functional changes in brain in an idiopathic headache syndrome. Nat Med 1999; 5(7): 836–838.

[21] Leone M, Proietti Cecchini A. Deep brain stimulation in headache. Cephalalgia 2015-in press.

[22] Leone M, Franzini A, Broggi G, Bussone G. Hypothalamic stimulation for intractable cluster headache: long-term experience. Neurology 2006; 67: 150–152.

[23] Bartsch T, Pinsker MO, Rasche D, Kinfe T, Hertel F, Diener HC, Tronnier V, Mehdorn HM, Volkmann J, Deuschl G, Krauss JK. Hypothalamic deep brain stimulation for cluster headache—experience from a new multicase series. Cephalalgia 2008; 28: 285–295.

[24] Fontaine D, Lazorthes Y, Mertens P, Blond S, Géraud G, Fabre N, Navez M, Lucas C, Dubois F, Gonfrier S, Paquis P, Lantéri-Minet M. Safety and efficacy of deep brain stimulation in refractory cluster headache: a randomized placebo controlled double-blind trial followed by a 1-year open extension. J Headache Pain 2010; 11: 23–31.

[25] Schoenen J, Di Clemente L, Vandenheede M, Fumal A, De Pasqua V, Mouchamps M, Remacle JM, de Noordhout AM. Hypothalamic stimulation in chronic cluster headache: a pilot study of efficacy and mode of action. Brain 2005; 128: 940–947.

[26] Seijo F, Saiz A, Lozano B, Santamarta E, Alvarez-Vega M, Seijo E, Fernández de León R, Fernández-González F, Pascual J. Neuromodulation of the posterolateral hypothalamus for the treatment of chronic refractory cluster headache: experience in five patients with a modified anatomical target. Cephalalgia 2011; 31: 1634–1641.

Section 2

From Bench to Bedside: What a Neurosurgeon Should Know

Chapter 4

Surgical Techniques in Benign Extra-Axial Tumors

Mario Ammirati and Alba Scerrati

Additional information is available at the end of the chapter

http://dx.doi.org/10.5772/64220

Abstract

Extra-axial tumors are lesions, neoplastic and not, which are external to the brain parenchyma and can originate in the skull, meninges, cranial nerves, and brain appendages such as the pituitary gland. Surgery provides a diagnosis and can be the first step in the treatment. When chosen as a treatment, we should consider the access and the approach to the lesion, the adequate operative technique, and related skills, minor or major complications. Because of the benign nature of these tumors, the evaluation of the risk/benefit in submitting a patient to a surgical treatment has to be considered. We would like to give an overview about benign extra-axial tumors and surgical operative techniques and tools that can be applied to improve patient's outcome.

Keywords: benign extra-axial tumors, surgical techniques, meningiomas, schwannomas, surgical approaches

1. Introduction and background

1.1. Definition, pathophysiology, and epidemiology

Extra-axial tumors are lesions, neoplastic and not, which are external to the brain parenchyma and can originate in the skull, meninges, cranial nerves, and brain appendages such as the pituitary gland. From a surgical point of view, it is important to understand their relationship with the subarachnoid spaces because it is in this space that nerves and vessels travel to and from the brain; hence, avoiding injury to these structures rests on a clear understanding of their relationships with the tumor. Lesions that originate outside the dura such as chordomas, chondrosarcomas, and paragangliomas are easy to understand as they are usually separated from neurovascular structures by an intact arachnoidal membrane.

Pituitary adenomas are intradural but extra-arachnoidal lesions. Meningiomas and cranial nerve schwannomas are usually covered by an arachnoidal layer but from a surgical point of view are extra-arachnoidal lesions, while epidermoid, dermoid, and craniopharingiomas are intra-arachnoidal and in the case of craniopharyngiomas occasionally intrapial lesions [1, 2].

They represent about one-third of all intracranial primary neoplasms in adults and about one-quarter of brain tumors in children [3].

They can be classified according to their site in supratentorial and infratentorial tumors.

The most common benign extra-axial lesions are meningiomas, pituitary adenomas, craniopharyngiomas, and cranial nerve schwannomas.

1.2. Clinical presentation

Because of their slow growth, the onset of symptoms can be insidious.

Supratentorial tumors can present with progressive focal deficits, mental status changes, or seizures. Infratentorial tumors can present with decreased hearing, gait disturbances, ataxia, vertigo, diplopia, multiple cranial nerves deficit, and long-tract abnormalities (if there is a brain stem involvement).

Common symptoms of both supratentorial and infratentorial masses are headache, nausea, and vomiting due to the increased intracranial pressure (ICP) [4, 5].

1.3. Diagnosis and imaging

Radiological imaging is of primary importance for a preoperative diagnosis.

Computerized tomography (CT) scan, without and with contrast, is usually the first diagnostic step and it can provide a better identification of tumors involving the bone and the presence of calcification.

Magnetic resonance imaging (MRI) is considered the gold standard because it provides a greater resolution for soft tissues and better identifies the margins and extent of the tumor, its relationship with nerves and vessels, and also affords optimal imaging of lesions about the skull base. Imaging features that are consistent with a benign tumor are usually homogeneous enhancement, smooth-rounded margins, no associated brain edema, and no satellite lesions.

Rising numbers of MRI studies performed during evaluations for different diseases caused a significant increase in the number of incidentally found brain tumors.

Conventional cerebral angiography is at times useful in the preoperative management of patients with meningiomas, occasionally for embolization purposes and more often to ascertain the patency of major sinuses and the alternative venous drainage when the lesion abuts or involves major dural sinuses [6].

1.4. Treatment options and alternatives

Different factors, patient and tumor related, are involved in the decision-making process. They can influence the possibility and extent of surgical resection or the choice of a nonsurgical treatment.

Factors can be classified as follows:

- Patient factors: neurologic conditions, comorbidities, age, and life expectancy;
- Tumor factors: location, size, vascular and neural involvement, and, in cases of recurrence, prior surgery or radiation therapy.

Conservative approach is based on monitoring the patient clinically and with serial MRI scans. It can be proposed for asymptomatic tumors (including incidental findings) with no evidence of growth or in elderly people with a high surgical risk [7, 8].

Age is becoming more and more of a relative concept with many papers demonstrating the safety of surgery—when indicated—in elderly people [9].

Surgery provides a diagnosis and can be the first step in the treatment.

Tumor excision improves symptoms related to increased intracranial pressure or those related to brain parenchyma/cranial nerves compression. When choosing surgery as a treatment, we should consider the access and the approach to the lesion, involvement of major vessels or cranial nerves, and risks for potential postoperative minor or major complications. Because of the benign nature of these tumors, the evaluation of the risk/benefit of a total resection versus a subtotal resection will be guided by the basic principle of "do no harm". Whenever a total resection presents a significant risk of morbidity (such as a neurological deficit or a fatal bleeding), part of the tumor can be left in situ and the patient can be submitted to clinical and radiological follow-up and eventually to surgery or focused beam radiation therapy in single or multiple fractions if tumors start re-growing or symptoms progress.

In cases where surgery is medically contraindicated, technically difficult, or high risk, primary radiation therapy may be considered as a definitive treatment option [10].

Radiation therapy for residual benign neoplasms is still somewhat controversial, although there is good evidence that subtotal excision plus radiotherapy produces local control and overall survival that is superior to subtotal removal alone. Timing of radiation therapy in cases of subtotal resection of a benign neoplasm is also somehow controversial with some authors using it only if and when there is evidence of tumor progression. The problem of arachnoid scarring created by radiotherapy makes reoperation for recurrence much more challenging. This concern needs to be balanced against the risk of earlier recurrence.

Finally, medical treatment can be considered for prolactinomas, who usually have a good response to dopamine agonist such as bromocriptine or cabergoline. For meningiomas, chemotherapies and hormonal therapies have been limited for the treatment of tumors that recur after surgery and when radiotherapy options are exhausted [11, 12]. They are considered generally ineffective, although somatostatin analogs may have therapeutic potential. There is also increasing interest in targeted molecular therapies. Agents inhibiting platelet-derived growth factor receptors and epidermal growth factor receptors have shown little efficacy, but molecular agents inhibiting vascular endothelial growth factor receptors appear to have some promise [13].

Although interest in pharmacotherapies against vestibular schwannoma is increasing [14], none are Food and Drug Administration (FDA) approved [15].

1.5. Goal and advantages of selected surgical approaches

When choosing a surgical approach, several considerations come into play:

- Exposure of the tumor and its margins, of its main arterial feeders, of its venous drainage and of the adjacent neurovascular structures. Clearly in large tumors all of these goals are unattainable;
- Adequate operative space to comfortably perform surgical maneuvers;
- Exposure of the lesions from multiple angles so as to be able to use different surgical corridors as needed;
- Minimize violation/trauma of the normal cerebral parenchyma at the expense of bone or extra-cerebral tissues removal;
- Respect as much as possible patient's aesthetics.

1.6. Indications

Indications for surgical treatment are as follows:

- Symptoms attributable to tumor compression of nearby structures;
- Demonstrated growth with sequential scans;
- Significant peritumoral edema;
- Need for diagnosis.

1.7. Contraindications

- High surgical risk related to the patient's age, clinical status, and comorbidities;
- Small asymptomatic tumors with no evidence of growth.

2. Operative details and preparation

2.1. Preoperative planning and special equipment

Good surgical results are not just dependent on surgeon's ability and skills but also on an accurate preoperative planning.

http://dx.doi.org/10.5772/64220

The side and site of the tumor and patient position has to be communicated to the operating room personnel in advance to properly position instruments and equipment before patient's arrival. Thromboembolism of the lower limbs has to be prevented using elastic or pneumatic stockings. Intraoperative-evoked potential, electroencephalogram, or other specialized monitoring devices are required in selected surgeries.

Navigation systems are helpful in planning skin and bone flaps, and in showing the relationships of the tumor to the bone and neurovascular structures of the skull base. When using neuronavigation for microsurgery of skull base tumors, the hand-held pointer needs to be replaced by the microscope/navigation integration where the microscope focal point becomes the tip of the virtual pointer. Indeed, using hand-held pointers is cumbersome and is not conducive to a smooth flow of the operation.

In selected cases, when cranial nerves or eloquent areas are involved by the tumor, intraoperative stimulation in and around a tumor will identify the functional tissue, and its preservation will minimize the risk of permanent postoperative deficit. In that regard, facial nerve stimulation in vestibular schwannoma surgery is fundamental in maximizing the chances of facial nerve preservation and functional integrity. It is important to remember that cranial nerve monitoring is only as good and helpful as the person who is able to read their traces and to critically interpret their changes as not to have under- or over-readings.

The role of endoscopic-assisted microsurgery relies on the seminal work of Perneczsky [16] and on the often-quoted sentence that "endoscopes allow visualization around the corners". While it is possible to introduce the endoscope in a microneurosurgical environment at the present time, its use may be made more efficient by the development and refining of good-quality display of the endoscopic image in the microscope oculars.

2.2.1. Microsurgical instruments

- Bipolar coagulation: the coagulation is localized and causes no current spread or radiation of heat to the surrounding tissues. The size, shape, weight, and balance of the bipolar forceps are important features of their design. A bayonet shape allows a better field of vision avoiding the block of the surgeon's hand. Bipolar forceps can also be used for dissection.

- Retractors: brain retraction has to be both minimized and properly used to prevent injuries. However, sometimes self-retaining retractors are useful to improve operative surgical angles or to reach deeper locations. Blades of different widths may be needed depending on the site and size of the lesion. One or more retractor blades are attached to a flexible arm near the resection site. Once the blade is on the desired position, the arm can be tightened. Retractor placement is a technical skill that needs to be mastered.

- Suction: the tip has to be smooth and atraumatic. The suction tube can also be used as a retractor or for a blunt dissection. Different diameters and lengths are available to better fit the depth and size of the surgical field.

- Tumor knives and forceps.

- Scissors: with fine blades on straight and bayonet handles are frequently used. Cutting should be done by the distal half of the blade. The blades can be straight or curved.
- Dissectors: divided in macro- and microdissector. Straight, rather than bayonet, dissectors are preferred for most intracranial operations because rotating the handles of the straight dissector does not alter the position of the tip. For transsphenoidal surgery, dissectors with bayonet handles are preferred because the surgeon's hand is prevented from blocking the view [17]. Different kinds of microdissector are as follows: round, spatula, flat, and micro-Penfield, nerve hook, angled and straight needle dissectors, microcurette, and teardrop dissectors.

Ultrasonic aspirators present the advantage to rapidly debulk tumors. Thanks to ultrasound waves, they fragment and aspirate tumor tissue. Care must be taken because they can quickly open through the surface of a tumor capsule and damage contiguous nerves and vessels.

Carbon dioxide laser produces energy that vaporizes tissues containing fluid. Because the beam cannot pass through fluid, its maximal effect is on the surface [17]. It is mainly used to debulk large tumors.

2.2.2. Microsurgical concepts: expert suggestions/comments

The key point in the removal of benign extra-axial neoplasm is the preservation of the arachnoidal plane that separate the tumor from the subarachnoid space and from the neurovascular structures contained in it. In the majority of cases, this plane may be preserved and at the end of the surgical procedures an intact layer of arachnoid where the tumor was may be recognized. To accomplish this key step, it is necessary to identify the tumor arachnoid interface. In large tumor, this may only be accomplished once the tumor size has been significantly decreased by internal (intracapsular) decompression (debulking) [1, 5].

Centripetal retraction of the tumor, away from the brain, rather than retract the brain parenchyma away from the tumor is considered another mainstay of microsurgical dissection.

The arachnoid must be grabbed with medium-size bayonet forceps and gently lifted off away from the tumor. The use of microbayonet, which are sharper than macrobayonet, will inevitably lead to violation of this interface. The use of curved tumor dissectors is helpful in further developing this plane even in areas that are not directly visualized, provided that the surgeon’s hand recognizes and properly interprets the proprioceptive feedbacks coming from the distal end of the instrument. Once separation has been accomplished, cottonoids of different sizes are introduced in the space created to maintain and identify it. Bipolar coagulation at this interface needs to be minimized because coagulation coalesces this interface and makes impossible atraumatic development of this plan. En bloc resection of large-size tumor is often impossible and dangerous; en bloc resection of medium-size tumor while tempting must be resisted for the sake of the principles discussed above. Annoying oozing from some area of the tumor may be controlled with topical hemostatic agents and gentle cottonoid applications while the attention of the surgeon goes to another area of the surgical field. Much has been made of early devascularization of large meningiomas; however, in many cases the main vascular pedicle is not accessible at the early stage of an intracranial procedure, and misguided attempts at accomplishing it may result in undue brain damage, often due to retraction. Meticulous attention has to be paid to all veins and attempts need to be made to preserve them, no matter their size.

Gentle retraction of the brain is one of the decisive general factors in minimizing postoperative complications. Again, brain retraction is a skill that needs to be mastered and studied. In general, it is better to work in a channel that is kept open by a properly placed retractor than to use in-and-out suction retraction. Positioning, administration of diuretics, drainage of cerebrospinal fluid (CSF), and hyperventilation are commonly used techniques that can help in reducing brain retraction. When the brain has to be retracted continuously, the retractor should be moved every few minutes to another part of the cortical surface or released for a while.

For tumors with potential involvement of the venous sinuses and draining veins, a preoperative MR venography or angiography will help the surgeon decide whether total excision is possible and which vessels can be sacrificed.

Microvascular Doppler can be used to localize major arteries that clearly need to be spared.

2.3. Key steps of the procedure

2.3.1. Patient positioning

When choosing the patient position, the following criteria have to be considered:

- Safety: the patient has to be secured and prevented from falling if the operating table needs to be moved during the surgery;
- Body compression sites have to be carefully inspected and protected with soft materials;
- Venous drainage has to be guaranteed: always place the head on higher level than the heart and avoid neck flexing that compresses jugular veins;
- Skin incision has to be completely visible and accessible;
- Gravity helps in brain relaxation.

2.3.2. Skin incision

When choosing the skin incision, the following criteria have to be considered:

- Maximal tumor exposure in the center of the surgical field minimizing the risk of injury to the surrounding neurovascular structures. Best results can be achieved with the use of neuronavigation.
- Vascular supply to the skin flap: in a wide flap, the base of the skin incision has to be proportional to its height. Careful evaluation of previous skin incision that can alter the normal vascularization of the skin flap is required.
- Avoidance of visible cosmetic defects.

2.3.3. Tumor excision

- To decide the craniotomy and the dural opening, neuronavigation can be used. The tumor has to be exposed as much as possible, minimizing normal brain parenchyma exposure. If there is cerebral edema, a wide bone and dural opening prevent cerebral compression and damage.
- Tumor devascularization has to be performed in the first stages whenever possible. It helps in reducing the blood loss and guarantees an easier tumor removal.
- General microneurosurgical concepts (already discussed) have to be followed.

2.3.4. Hemostasis

When the tumor excision has ended, the hemostasis of the surgical field has to be very accurate to prevent postoperative bleeding.

The following steps need to be followed:

- Generous washing of the surgical cavity to remove all blood clots;
- Bipolar coagulation of all the active bleeding points;
- Avetin is microfibrillar bovine collagen that favors the platelet aggregation at the site of oozing. It is helpful in control oozing from raw brain parenchyma. Flowseal ,Gelfoam, and Surgicel may also be used;
- Once hemostasis has been achieved, perform a Valsalva maneuver to make sure there is no occult bleeding;
- Dural suspensions to control epidural bleeding.

2.3.5. Closure

The dura has to be closed to avoid CSF leaks. If the patient dura is not available, galea or synthetic dural substitutes can be used.

A 4-0-silk stitches can be used to perform a continuous suture. At the end, fibrin glue can be spread all over the dura to increase the sealing. An onlay Duragen or a similar material may be used to reinforce the dural closure.

The bone can be fixed with titanium screws and plates. If the patient's bone is not available, bone substitutes can be used.

Muscle reconstruction is very important. In frontotemporal approaches, the temporal muscle has to be reconstructed properly to avoid mastication problems and cosmetic defects. In posterior fossa muscle layers reconstruction represents a further barrier for CSF leaks.

Management of intracranial air containing spaces: if the frontal sinus mucosa is violated, then complete exenterating of the frontal sinus and its mucosa is usually recommended. The nasofrontal ducts are plugged with fat and fibrin glue. A more generous fat graft may be needed if a large dead space is present or to supplement the dural closure when needed. Entered mastoid cells are plugged with bone wax, fat, and fibrin glue.

Skin flap has to be properly closed to avoid subcutaneous haemorrhages, CSF leaks, and cosmetic defects.

2.4. Surgical approaches

For supratentorial tumors, the most common approaches are as follows:

- Monolateral or bilateral subfrontal approaches: for the access to the anterior cranial fossa and anterior midline structures, posterior orbit and apex [18], the bifrontal approach is preferred when treating larger or purely midline lesions because of its better angle of view. When dealing with tumors such as olfactory groove meningiomas, a direct access to anterior ethmoid arteries is possible. Their coagulation reduces the dural blood supply to these lesions. Moreover, the position of the head in the subfrontal approaches reduces the intraoperative brain retraction taking advantage of gravity. The use of lumbar drain is often helpful when dealing with large lesions that preclude early access to CSF spaces.

- Frontotemporal/pterional approach: for tumors located in the anterior and middle cranial fossa, in the sphenoid, parasellar, and cavernous sinus regions, this approach forms a pyramidal-shaped working space whose apex is directed toward the limen insulae [1]. Splitting the Sylvian fissure allows the frontal lobe to fall away from the temporal lobe with minimal or no retraction. Early brain relaxation can be achieved opening the basal cisterns. The pterional approach allows the access and control of vital structures such as carotid artery and its main branches, cranial nerves, and the cavernous sinus region.

- Fronto-orbito-zygomatic approach: it offers a wide angle of exposure and a greater rostral trajectory for the management of lesions involving the cavernous sinus, parasellar region, upper clivus, and adjacent neurovascular structures. Removing the zygomatic arch enables the temporalis muscle to be displaced inferiorly, allowing a better subtemporal visualization. However, one should keep in mind that the periorbita is an unyielding structure that should not be unduly compressed. Hence, the advantage of removing the orbital roof is marginal.

- Basal interhemispheric approach: for tumors of the sagittal midline arising deep to the flax.

- Transsphenoidal approach: for pathologies involving the sella, suprasellar space, and sphenoid bone. It provides excellent visualization of the pituitary and is minimally traumatic to the brain, and avoids brain retraction and visible scars. It can be performed by the use of an operative microscope (with the advantage of a three-dimensional (3D) viewing) or by an endoscope (who enlarges the surgeon's field of view).

For infratentorial tumors, the most common approaches are as follows:

- Suboccipital median/paramedian/lateral approach: for tumors located in the posterior fossa and cerebello-pontine angle (CPA). The suboccipital lateral approach gives access to the CPA and allows early identification of various neurovascular structures. The surgical exposure extends from the trigeminal nerve and tentorium superiorly to the foramen magnum and jugular foramen inferiorly [19].

- Far lateral approach: for tumors located in the vertebro-basilar junction. Adding a C1 laminectomy to the standard suboccipital craniectomy provides adequate visualization of approximately 270° of the circumference around the medulla.
- Subtemporal and Kawase's approach: for tumors located in the middle fossa and in the petroclival region. It provides a lower manipulation of cranial nerves. Adding the anterior petrosectomy gives access to the internal acoustic meatus and both middle and posterior fossa. Surgical adjuncts such as division of the tentorium and zygomatic osteotomy can provide additional working space and versatility.
- Translabyrinthine or transcochlear petrosal approach: for tumors located in the CPA, when hearing is already compromised. It gives a wide exposure and surgical space, avoiding cerebellar retraction.

2.5. Avoidances/hazards/risks

When choosing a surgical treatment, we should consider its indications and the balance of associated risks and reasonable goals. When considering hazards and risks, patient factors such as age, life expectancy, neurologic condition, and general medical conditions should be taken into account. In addition, tumor factors should be considered. Higher risks include the following:

- Location: tumor located close to eloquent areas;
- Infiltration of dural sinuses;
- Infiltration of major arteries;
- Cranial nerve involvement.

2.6. Salvage and rescue

It is important to have a clear preoperative plan. However, more important is the ability to modify the preoperative plan based on the operative findings. Indeed, it is impossible to know preoperatively what is the tumor consistency, which is a major determinant, everything else being equal, of the challenges associated with its removal. It is important to keep in mind that the majority, the overwhelming majority of extra-axial tumors, have a benign clinical course and that most of them respond to focused radiotherapy, in single or multiple fractions.

3. Outcomes and postoperative course

3.1. Complications

Postoperative fastidious patient monitoring can detect early complications.

http://dx.doi.org/10.5772/64220

In general, increasing headache in the postoperative period should not be treated symptomatically unless and until a postoperative complication has been ruled out by a CT/MRI.

These are the most common complications and their management:

- Bleeding:
  - in the tumor bed;
  - Subdural;
  - Epidural;
  - Subcutaneous.

  The management strictly depends on the entity of the bleeding and on the compression on the brain parenchyma or neurovascular structures. The patient can be clinically or radiologically monitored or may need a surgical evacuation of the hematoma.

- CSF leaks: more common in posterior fossa approaches. A conservative management consists of wound medication and a spinal CSF drainage placement. If the leak still persists, there is a higher risk of infection and surgery with a wound revision has to be performed.
- Infections: patients with CSF leaks, or comorbidities, present a higher risk. The infection can involve just the superficial layers and in these cases it can be managed by an antibiotic therapy. If the bone, dura, or the surgical field is involved, a surgical wound revision is needed.
- Neurological deficits: they can be caused by brain parenchyma injury, edema or ischemia (for a vessel occlusion), or by cranial nerves damage. The management is conservative in most of the case with anti-edema therapy and brain protection. The neurological deficit can be temporary and the patient can recover in few months. If there is a persistent damage to the facial nerve, a hypoglossofacial nerve anastomosis can be indicated.
- Deep vein thrombosis (DVT) and pulmonary embolism: higher risk for patients who develop neurological deficit or present a complicated postoperative course. Treatment is based on anticoagulant therapy. In cases of a massive pulmonary embolism, an endovascular treatment can be indicated.

3.2. Outcomes and prognosis

Outcomes depend on the kind of tumor and its location, on the kind of removal (if total or subtotal), and on the presence of intraoperative or postoperative complications.

Since these are benign tumors, prognosis is good in most of the cases and can be little modified by the amount of surgical excision.

Author details

Mario Ammirati[1*] and Alba Scerrati[2]

*Address all correspondence to: Mario.Ammirati@osumc.edu

1 The Ohio State University Wexner Medical Center, Columbus, OH, USA

2 Catholic University of Rome, Rome, Italy

References

[1] Yasargil GM. Operative anatomy in Microneurosurgery. Vol. 1.Pag.14. Thieme Stratton, 1984 ISBN0865771413, 9780865771413.

[2] Ciric I1, Rosenblatt S, Zhao JC. Transsphenoidal microsurgery. Neurosurgery. 2002 Jul; 51(1):161–9 (pub-id: 12182414)

[3] Osborne AG. Extra-Axial Neoplasms, Cysts and Tumor-like lesions. In Gourtsoyiannis NC, Ros PR, ed. Radiologic-Pathologic Correlations from Head to Toe. Understanding the Manifestations of Disease. Pag.27–33.Springer-Verlag Berlin Heidelberg 2005 ISBN 978-3-540-26664-8.

[4] Greenberg MS. Brain Tumors – General Clinical Aspects . In Greenberg MS, ed. Handbook of Neurosurgery.(pag. 404–405) Thieme; 6 edition (2004).

[5] Ammirati M, Zarzour H. Overview of Skull Base Tumors. In Win HR, ed. Youmann's Neurological Surgery. Vol. 2.6th ed. (pag. 1569–1586) Philadelphia, PA : Saunders/ Elsevier, 2011.

[6] Cernov M, DeMonte F. Skull Base Tumors. In Levin VA, ed. Cancer in the Nervous System. 2nd ed. Oxford University Press 2003.

[7] Jadid KD, Feychting M, Höijer J, Hylin S, Kihlström L, Mathiesen T. Long-term follow-up of incidentally discovered meningiomas. Acta Neurochir (Wien). 2015 Feb;157(2): 225–30 (pub-id: 25503298).

[8] Stangerup SE, Caye-Thomasen P, Tos M, Thomsen J. The natural history of vestibular schwannoma. Otol Neurotol. 2006 Jun;27(4):547–52 (pub-id: 16791048).

[9] Chen ZY, Zheng CH, Tang Li, Su XY, Lu GH, Zhang CY, Xiao SW, Tan YF. Intracranial meningioma surgery in the elderly (over 65 years): prognostic factors and outcome. Acta Neurochir (Wien). 2015 Sep;157(9):1549–57; discussion 1557 (pub-id: 26170189).

[10] Berger MS, Prados MD. Treatment Principles. In Berger MS, Prados MD, ed. Texbook of Neuroncology, pag.342.Saunders; 1 edition 2004.

[11] McMullen KP, Stieber VW. Meningioma: current treatment options and future directions. Curr Treat Options Oncol. 2004 Dec;5(6):499–509 (pub-id:15509483).

[12] Sioka C, Kyritsis AP. Chemotherapy, hormonal therapy, and immunotherapy for recurrent meningiomas. J Neurooncol. 2009 Mar;92(1):1–6 (pub-id:19023520).

[13] Wen PY, Quant E, Drappatz J, Beroukhim R, Norden AD. Medical therapies for meningiomas. J Neurooncol. 2010 Sep;99(3):365–78 (pub-id: 20820875).

[14] Plotkin SR, Merker VL, Halpin C, Jennings D, McKenna MJ, Harris GJ, Barker FG. Bevacizumab for progressive vestibular schwannoma in neurofibromatosis type 2: a retrospective review of 31 patients. Otol Neurotol. 2012 Aug;33(6):1046–52 (pub-id: 22805104).

[15] Dilwali S, Briët MC, Kao SY, Fujita T, Landegger LD, Platt MP, Stankovic KM. Preclinical validation of anti-nuclear factor-kappa B therapy to inhibit human vestibular schwannoma growth. Mol Oncol. 2015 Aug;9(7):1359–70 (pub-id: 25891780).

[16] Perneczky A, Fries G. Endoscope-assisted brain surgery: part 1 evolution, basic concept, and current technique. Neurosurgery. 1998 Feb;42(2):219–24; discussion 224–5 (pub-id: 9482171).

[17] Rhoton AL Jr. General Principles of and Instrumentation for Cranial Surgery. In Fessler RG, Sekhar LN, ed. Atlas of Neurosurgical Techniques, pag. 3–42. Thieme; 1 edition, 2006.

[18] Kawakami K, Yamanouchi Y, Kubota C, Kawamura Y, Matsumura H. An extensive transbasal approach to frontal skull-base tumors: technical note. J Neurosurg 1991;74:1011–3 (pub-id: 2033437).

[19] Mostafa BE, El Sharnoubi M, Youssef AM. The keyhole retrosigmoid approach to the cerebello-pontine angle: indications, technical modifications, and results. Skull Base. 2008 Nov;18(6):371–6.

Chapter 5

Lumbar Spinal Stenosis, Clinical Presentation, Diagnosis, and Treatment

Luiz Cláudio Lacerda Rodrigues

Additional information is available at the end of the chapter

http://dx.doi.org/10.5772/63920

Abstract

Lumbar spinal stenosis (LSS), a disease that mainly affects people over 50 years old, may have a dramatic presentation with pain, difficulty in walking, changes in urinary functions in addition to root symptoms, such as numbness, burning, and feeling of heaviness in the legs. The treatment is very varied with several non-surgical and surgical possibilities. With an aging population, this disease becomes increasingly preoccupant for their uncertain evolution and without a well-defined correlation with imaging tests, treatment, and outcome may be troublesome. Moreover, LSS frequently affects patients who have associated comorbidity that can hinder the treatment.

Keywords: lumbar stenosis, outcomes, degenerative disc, pathophysiology, surgical treatment, non-surgical treatment

1. Introduction

Lumbar canal stenosis was first described by Antoine Portal in 1803. However, Verbiest [1, 2] was the first to associate changes in the diameter of the vertebral canal with the clinical features and neurogenic claudication. The reduced canal diameter was only correlated to the disc degenerative process by Kirkaldy-Willis, when the authors demonstrated that disc degeneration was directly related to the changes that lead to the physiopathology of reduced vertebral canal diameter [3].

Based on a study of dissection of 50 cadavers, Kirkaldy and Willis described how changes in the zygapophyseal joints and disc degeneration may lead to root impingement and, consequently, all the set of symptoms, which will be discussed in depth later [4].

According to Farfan [5], the degenerative process starts with minor trauma, which, repeated over several years, leads to spondylosis. A few years later, Farfan et al. [6] described how each segment of the lumbar spine is composed of a complex triad: two zygapophyseal joints and the disc. Because those three joints work in tandem, any disease that affects the disc will eventually compromise the joint and vice versa. The chief lesion mechanisms are torsional forces and compression overload [7].

Farfan also describes how the degenerative process starts between the fourth and fifth lumbar vertebrae and that after that level is compromised, based on the three-joint theory, the degeneration progresses to the proximal and distal adjacent levels. Thus, it becomes a diffuse disease that affects multiple levels of the lumbar spine. The anatomic changes are described next.

The zygapophyseal joints are diarthrodial, having an articular surface, a synovial membrane, and a capsule made of collagen; they are filled with synovial fluid [8]. Their degenerative process follows a sequence described by Lewin in 1964 [9]: it starts with a synovial reaction, followed by fibrillation of the joint surface, gross degeneration of the cartilage, osteophyte formation, joint process fracture, and finally loss of the joint's natural shape, leading to instability.

The third component of this complex joint is the intervertebral disc, the largest nonvascular tissue in the human body [10], which comprises three structures: the nucleus pulposus, the annulus fibrosus, and the terminal plates [3]. Each one of these structures has its own anatomy and unique constitution, and considerable importance [10]. The annulus fibrosus is made of type I collagen, distributed in circular layers, and resistant to traction forces. The nucleus pulposus is made basically of proteoglycans, water, and type II collagen, as well as countless elastin fibers [11]. Nutrition of the disc cells occurs through diffusion, in which vessels in the subchondral space, adjacent to the terminal plate's hyaline cartilage, carry oxygen, glucose, and small molecules, thus maintaining the disc's homeostasis [12]. Such homeostasis allows the nucleus pulposus to withstand compressive forces without collapsing and forces to be homogeneously transferred to the annulus fibrosus in all spine movements [13].

Another anatomic area that may go unnoticed is the lateral region, including the intervertebral foramen. Lee et al. [14] subdivided this region into three zones: the afferent zone, located in the subarticular region, medially to the pedicles; the intermediate or middle zone, located below the pars interarticularis; and finally, the efferent zone, comprising the intervertebral foramen. The latter is very important in surgical cases, because a lack of identification may lead to incorrect decompression and persistence of symptoms after surgery [15]. The foramen is a relatively large orifice, which often contains the dorsal root ganglion, coated with a layer of fat for the protection of neural structures. It is delimited anteriorly by the posterior vertebral wall, proximally by the inferior edge of the superior pedicle, inferiorly by the superior edge of the inferior pedicle, and posteriorly by the zygapophyseal joints and the yellow ligament.

2. Historical Background

The degenerative process can also be observed in this region, where diffuse disc bulging can also be seen, associated with loss of height—all leading to a reduced diameter of the vertebral canal. The zygapophyseal joints are also directly associated with foramen stenosis, because their hypertrophy may or may not be associated with the presence of osteophytes, thus causing radicular compression. In this case, sciatica may be observed, mimicking the symptoms of disc herniation [16].

The progression of the degenerative disease still remains truly unknown [17]. However, many concepts have already been postulated. The first one concerns the definition of instability; it is defined as "excessive mobility, neural compression, or deformity." The presence of instability may be associated with a variety of clinical and anatomic manifestations [18].

Kirkaldy and Willis described the degenerative process in terms of evolution and divided it into three phases. However, the duration of each stage is unknown. The first phase was described as a dysfunction in which the disc exhibits chiefly biochemical changes. The second phase was called instability in which degenerative processes in the disc lead to an increase in the segment's motion; this is when disc herniation can occur. Finally, there is the stabilization phase in which disc height reduction, facet hypertrophy, and changes in the yellow ligament occur [18]. This phase of disc degeneration is the most important for the development of the present study, because the aforementioned changes lead to a reduction of the vertebral canal diameter and to narrow lumbar spinal canal syndrome—the disease that is the object of this study.

As was described by Kirkaldy and Willis, the cascading degeneration does not have a definite phase, but in the stabilization phase, lumbar canal stenosis can be observed. It may or may not cause symptoms, but if symptoms do occur, this is commonly observed in patients above 50 years of age. Currently, the most commonly performed type of spine surgery in patients over 65 years old in the United States is decompression of cauda equina roots [19].

Because the population is aging and life expectancy is increasing, we were motivated to conduct this project.

Narrow lumbar spinal canal syndrome comprises a number of symptoms and varied clinical features [20], which is further discussed below.

Vertebral canal stenosis, as defined by Verbiest [2], corresponds to narrowing of the vertebral canal, the lateral recess, and the intervertebral foramen, causing compression of neural elements. Vertebral canal stenosis can be divided into two main groups: congenital and acquired [21]. These main groups were further subdivided: congenital stenosis into idiopathic and achondroplasic, and acquired stenosis into degenerative, combined, spondylotic, iatrogenic, post-traumatic, and metabolic [21].

Narrow lumbar spinal canal syndrome may be confused with many other diseases. Such diseases must always be considered, and a detailed clinical examination may make all the difference. Among the conditions that should be investigated are disc herniation, vascular claudication, tumors, peripheral neuropathy, arthrosis of the hip or knee, and compressive insufficiency fractures [16].

Hall et al. [22] described symptomatic canal stenosis in detail. They described that patients complain of progressive lumbar pain, associated with an incipient pain and numbness in the distal extremities. Neurogenic claudication, the commonest symptom, is characterized by pain and weakness starting in the buttocks and thighs that becomes gradually worse in the orthostatic position and during walking, but improves after sitting down or leaning forward. Less often, one can find unilateral radiculopathy [23]. Symptoms become more acute with the disease's natural progression [24].

The progression of the disease is uncertain: according to Johnson, 70% of patients remain stable for a 4-year period, 15% improve, and 15% tend to become worse. The progression to cauda equina syndrome is extremely rare, but must always be investigated, particularly because of the possibility of other causes, but also because it is an absolute indication for urgent surgery [25].

Elderly patients may present a clinical condition very similar to neurogenic claudication, an entity called vascular claudication, associated with atherosclerosis. The pain following a walk is very similar to that in neurogenic claudication. Physical examination then becomes essential, because in a detailed examination, one can observe impotence in men, dystrophic skin, loss of hair, nail dystrophy, cyanosis, and reduced peripheral pulse. Such symptoms may be essential for the latter diagnosis [22].

3. Physical Examination

The best diagnostic test to distinguish both syndromes was described by Van Gelderen [26]. He had patients riding a stationary bicycle. Patients with lumbar canal stenosis tolerate the exercise, because the forward-leaning position causes symptoms to improve, whereas patients with vascular claudication do not tolerate the exercise, because the hypoxia caused by the underlying disease causes pain and peripheral cyanosis. Another very relevant sign in narrow canal syndrome is improvement when walking uphill and worsening when walking downhill, always associated with the flexion or extension of the trunk [27, 28]. It is postulated that the improvement associated with flexion and extension is directly related to stretching or folding of the yellow ligament. Trunk flexion causes tension in this ligament, thus increasing its diameter, whereas trunk extension causes it to fold into the spinal canal, thus further narrowing the canal that is already narrowed by the degenerative process [29, 30].

The physical examination of a patient with lumbar canal stenosis starts with the careful observation, followed by a very thorough physical examination. One must always consider the differential diagnosis from the other above-mentioned conditions; however, when compared to disc herniation, there are some subtle differences, such as age above 50 years, insidious onset, improvement with trunk flexion and worsening with its extension, and localized motor weakness. Signs of dura mater tension and muscular contraction are rarely found. Typically, a trunk flexion position is observed, due to the increased canal diameter in that position. The presence of a reduced arc of movement is associated with the joint's degenerative process and not directly with the lumbar canal stenosis. Analogous to Phalen's test, Kemp's test is described in the literature, in which the patient is kept in trunk extension for 30 s and claudication symptoms appear [31].

4. Diagnostic

Radiological diagnosis includes several examinations: common radiography, computed tomography (CT), and magnetic resonance imaging (MRI). In selected cases, myelography or myelotomography may be necessary [32].

The study of neural function and conduction speed can be performed either by electroneuromyography or by sensitive-motor evoked potentials [32].

Radiographs must be obtained in four incidences: frontal, orthostatic lateral, flexion, and extension. Then one must look for degenerative changes, such as reduced disc space, sclerosis of vertebral plateaus, sclerosis and hypertrophy of articular facets, closeness of spinous processes, and the diameter of the intervertebral foramina. In dynamic radiography, one can notice the presence of anteroposterior translation [33].

Computed tomography is a very important advance in the diagnosis of vertebral stenosis, because it shows important bone details, including the central canal, the lateral recess, the foramen, the joint facets, and their degree of degeneration [34]. CT is, however, criticized for its high rate of radiologic findings without correlation to the patient's symptoms [33].

MRI provides images of soft tissue with excellent quality, including ligaments, neural tissue, and the intervertebral discs. It is more sensitive for diagnosing lumbar stenosis than tomography. MRI findings include signal weakening at T2, with dehydration and rupture of the annulus in multiple discs; changes in terminal plates; void signal; enlarged yellow ligaments; and reduced vertebral canal [35].

For many years, myelography was the gold-standard exam for diagnosing lumbar stenosis, but although today's water-soluble contrast is less toxic, patients still have nausea, vomiting, headache, and dizziness. Myelography is an invasive exam, although it shows the dimensions of the dural sac and the neural roots in detail. Myelography findings include the partial or total interruption of contrast flow, and the dynamic examination may reveal a dynamic compression of neural structures [36]. It should be noted that electromyography is not routinely used in lumbar stenosis, because 80% of symptomatic patients have changes in one or both legs, making it necessary only for differential diagnosis, particularly to distinguish it from diseases that affect peripheral nerves [37].

The canal's diameter may be calculated by several different techniques. We used Hamanishi's technique, widely used [38], on which the calculation to determine the presence of stenosis is based. That is, Hamanishi considers a diameter of less than 100 mm^2 to define stenosis in patients with clinical symptoms and characteristic images [39].

The treatment of lumbar canal stenosis may be divided into two main types: clinical or conservative and surgical [40], each of them comprising several different modalities.

When a thorough clinical examination has been performed and there is confirmation from imaging exams, electrodiagnosis is not needed, as results are often inconclusive and, when positive, do not have an influence on either the clinical or the surgical treatment [41].

Generally, clinical treatment is preferred by over 50% of patients [42], and they mostly evolve satisfactorily. However, a small fraction suffers a more severe progression, with more unfavorable natural history and serious, limiting symptoms [43].

Many lumbar canal stenosis patients have symptoms of unilateral radiculopathy. In such cases, the most likely cause is herniation, which may affect a root in an already stenotic canal. When this happens, treatment should be more focused on the disc herniation. Despite the large number of articles in the literature, there is no consensus about when to operate such patients and, if surgery is performed, what the best technique would be [44].

5. Treatment Options

Drug treatment does not offer many possibilities. The indiscriminate and frequent use of anti-inflammatory medications for chronic lumbar pain does not have a proven satisfactory response [45] and may be associated with gastrointestinal and renal complications. Its use should be very restricted and avoided in elderly patients with narrow lumbar spinal canal syndrome [45].

Simple painkillers, muscle relaxants, and opioids may be of value. They are indicated for treating and controlling the pain but have no effect on the treatment of neurogenic claudication [45]. Gabapentin has been shown to be a safe medication; it may be taken orally and has a positive effect on patients with neurogenic claudication and the sensory alterations, which are very common in these patients [46].

Corticosteroids are also used indiscriminately. The idea is that there is an inflammatory process associated with the mechanical compression that could benefit from the medication, but this theory was not proven by Natour's study [47].

Physiotherapy, or more broadly rehabilitation, is a second non-surgical approach. Manual therapy, stretching, and muscular strengthening play an important role, in addition to the exercises. Patients who suffer from canal stenosis have, in addition to pain, a significant muscle loss, which severely limits their activities and progressively worsens their clinical condition, which leads to further impairments [48, 49].

The recommended activities include manual therapy, strengthening, and walking training, as well as exercises that improves proprioception. In addition, weight loss is important, because obese patients have been described to have a worse prognosis [47]. Cycling is a very much recommended activity, not only because patients tolerate it well, but it also allows them to improve their conditioning and does not impact other joints that may also be degenerated, such as the hip and the knee [50].

Zarife et al. [51], in a study comparing two types of conservative treatments—physiotherapy and peridural corticosteroids—concluded that, in a 6-month follow-up, both methods were effective in improving the patients' condition and ability to walk, which suggested that clinical treatment is important and effective in these delicate and active patients.

Peridural corticosteroids are another type of non-surgical treatment for narrow lumbar spinal canal syndrome, as opposed to oral corticosteroids, which were shown to be ineffective for this condition [47]. Peridural corticosteroids have some advantages, which are discussed below. There are several possibilities for their administration, with or without radioscopy, as well as several techniques: interlaminar, caudal, and transforaminal. Despite their limited benefits, their use may have lasting efficacy in many patients [52].

Cosgrove et al. [53] published an article in 2011 in which the efficacy of peridural corticosteroids was evaluated and showed that women obtained greater benefits than men and that clinical results were not related to MR findings, which was also found in Natour's study [47]. Although Cosgrove et al. [53] observed better results among women, as per the general literature, women are normally affected compared to men.

Similarly to the above-mentioned article, Charles et al. [54] showed that peridural corticosteroids produce a satisfactory response in lumbar stenosis. The results of the study showed that patients with associated radiculopathy have a better response than do patients with claudication and that 25% of patients respond more favorably up to 2 years after the procedure.

However, we also found some articles in which the use of peridural corticosteroids did not deliver the expected satisfaction, in addition to causing complications such as meningitis, arachnoiditis, aseptic meningitis, and increased serum corticosteroids [55]. Fukusaki et al. [56] compared the use of analgesics in isolation and in combination with peridural corticosteroids and reported no complications; however, the results after 3 months were unsatisfactory, with all symptoms returning.

Surgical treatment is considered the last resort for patients with treating lumbar canal stenosis. Because surgery is performed in patients over 65 years of age, there is significant morbidity and mortality, which increase with associated diseases and patient age, making it mandatory to assess the risks and benefit of the surgery [57].

Airaksinen's study [58] showed that patients over 50 years old who underwent decompression and arthrodesis evolved with a significantly reduced ability to return to work. That reduction was even greater in older patients.

There are articles that report surgical results, with conflicting results. Hurri et al. [59], in a 12-year follow-up study, did not find any differences between surgical and non-surgical results, showing that regardless of surgery, the outcome is the same. Another study comparing operated and non-operated patients was the Maine Lumbar Spine Study [60, 61], in which operated patients were followed up for a period from 4 to 10 years. Results showed that operated patients had better postoperative results than non-operated patients, with an average of 72% satisfaction among the former and 52% among the latter at 4 years of follow-up. The same comparison made at 10 years showed inferior results, but operated patients still had a perception of improvement.

Turner et al. [62] performed a meta-analysis and found that 64% of patients showed good results after surgical treatment, for a period varying from 3 to 6 years.

Surgical treatment is indicated when clinical treatment fails or neurological symptoms worsen [63]. Today, there are several different surgical techniques. The classical technique is laminectomy, performed by an incision along the midline followed by decompression, removing up to 50% of facets. In addition, there are minimally invasive techniques, such as opening and decompressing only one side of the lamina, which is called recalibration [64]. Interspinous spacers have been recently included in the surgical arsenal for canal stenosis, but studies are still under way, and there are no studies yet evaluating for an adequate follow-up period. For this reason, the actual benefit of this kind of surgery is not yet well established. However, it is known that it does offer some advantages, such as short hospitalization periods and limited bleeding. Its indication takes into account that by tensioning the yellow ligament, the canal diameter is increased [65].

The median approach with broad exposure of the spine has the advantage of satisfactorily exposing the spinal canal, which allows the intervertebral foramina to be viewed, broad decompression to happen up to the efferent zone with direct view, and roots to be evaluated. However, care must be taken to preserve half of the facets; otherwise, postoperative instability will occur as an iatrogenic complication that may compromise the results for the patient. The main problem with this broad approach is blood loss, which may be large or even catastrophic in some cases, because muscular lesion leads to large arterial and venous bleeding [63].

The indication for instrumentation and fusion varies in the literature, with some authors indicating fusion in the presence of degenerative spondylolisthesis or if there is a translation greater than 5 mm in dynamic X-rays. Instrumentation may also be indicated in cases of degenerative scoliosis in which the neural foramen is compressed on the concave side of the curvature and resection of more than 50% of the articular facet is needed in order to decompress the root stuck inside [66, 67].

The minimally invasive approach in spinal canal stenosis associated with foraminal stenosis may be indicated for patients with lumbar and radicular pain associated with stenosis in imaging exams, but its main contraindication is the presence of instability in X-rays, associated with a scoliosis of more than 10° in X-rays, in the orthostatic position. The main complication is recurring symptoms, in approximately 20% of cases, with reoperation being necessary, with broad exposure of the spine [68].

Interspinous spacers are a new generation of implants. Their mechanism of action is by blocking extension, as well as tensioning the stenosis level, which theoretically increases the spinal canal diameter. Studies have shown that such an increase may reach 20% of the initial diameter [69], but these studies are questioned due to the possibility of commercial interests. They are indicated for lumbar canal stenosis patients with two levels of stenosis, but they are not used in the L5-S1 level and are contraindicated for patients with degenerative spondylolisthesis or radiological signs of instability [70].

Postoperative care of lumbar canal stenosis patients may vary slightly, but basically, patients are instructed to walk on the first day after surgery. Longer rest is indicated for patients with incidental durotomy, in which case the recommendation is at least 2 days rest. Deambulation with the aid and training by a physiotherapist is very important [71]. Rehabilitation exercises must include stretching the posterior muscles of the thighs and legs, training trunk flexibility, and strengthening the abdominal and paravertebral muscles. Improving cardiopulmonary capacity is also a target of rehabilitation, always respecting the patients' limits [72].

The need for orthesis is very much relative. Their use is generally not indicated. In osteoporotic patients, when there is the risk of an acute failure of implants, their use may be indicated for a period of up to 6 weeks, but overall, the literature is highly controversial about this subject [73].

The complications observed in surgery for lumbar canal stenosis may be divided into complications in the operated area and systemic complications. The most commonly observed systemic complications are urinary retention, worsening of heart failure in previously affected patients, delirium, and thoracic pain. Such symptoms are usually temporary, but they increase hospitalization time [74].

Surgical complications vary according to the series. Jolles et al. [75] report sensorial and motor deficit, dura mater lesions with cerebrospinal fluid fistula, surgical site hematoma, and superficial and deep infection.

Epidemiologically, surgery for lumbar canal stenosis has the same incidence of complications as knee arthroplasties, but greater than hip arthroplasties [76]. Mortality is currently at an average of 10%, but it increases with patient age. Clinical complications vary from 3 to 31% [77]. However, the most common complication observed in lumbar canal stenosis surgery is incidental durotomy, with an average incidence of 16%, increasing in case of reoperation [78]. Cerebrospinal fluid fistula, with leakage of cerebrospinal fluid, is the chief cause of reoperation in the first 2 days after surgery [79].

6. Conclusion

In conclusion, lumbar canal stenosis is a complex syndrome, which comprises degenerative processes in the lumbar spine. This degeneration may lead to a painful and limiting clinical condition, which must always be investigated through an exhaustive study of imaging examinations. Even though treatment is varied, with a large number of possibilities found in the literature, studies usually compare different techniques, either surgical or conservative, to find the most effective one. Apparently, the surgical approach with decompression, either associated with arthrodesis or not, has provided not only the best clinical results but also a greater incidence of complications and mortality, which must always be weighed together with the patient before surgery.

Author details

Luiz Cláudio Lacerda Rodrigues

Address all correspondence to: luizclaudiolacerdarodrigues@gmail.com

1 Santa Marcelina Medical School, São Paulo, Brazil

2 Oswaldo Cruz German Hospital, Rua Treze de Maio, São Paulo - SP, Brazil

References

[1] Verbiest H. A radicular syndrome from developmental narrowing of the lumbar vertebral canal. J Bone Joint Surg Br;36:230–237, 1954.

[2] Verbiest H. The significance and principles of computerized axial tomography in idiopathic developmental stenosis of the bony lumbar vertebral canal. Spine;4:369–378, 1979.

[3] Kirkaldy-Willis WH, Paine KW, Cauchoix J, Mclvor G. Lumbar spinal stenosis. Clin Orthop;99:30–50, 1974.

[4] Kirkaly-Willis WH, Wedge JH, Yong-Hing K, Reilly J. Pathology and pathogenesis of lumbar spondylosis and stenosis. Spine;3(4):319–328, 1978.

[5] Farfan HF. Effects of torsion on the intervertebral joints. Can J Surg;12:336–341, 1969.

[6] Farfan HF, Sulivan JB. The relation of facet orientation to intervertebral disc failure. Can J Surg;10:179–18, 1967.

[7] Yong-Hing K, Reilly J, Kirkald-Willis WH. The ligamentun flavum. Spine;1:226–234, 1976.

[8] Sullivan JD, Farfan HF, Kahn DS. Pathological changes with intervertebral joint rotational instability in the rabbit. Can J Surg;13:71–79, 1971.

[9] Lewin T. Osteoartrits in lumbar synovial joints. Acta Orthop Scand Suple;73:1–112, 1964.

[10] Yong-soo C. Pathophysiology of degenerative disc disease. Asian Spine J;3(1):39–44, 2009.

[11] Borgesen SE, Vang PS. Herniation of the lumbar intervertebral disk in children and adolescents. Acta Orthop Scand;45:540–549, 1974.

[12] Key JA. Intervertebral disc lesions in children and adolescents. J Bone Joint Surg Am; 32:97–102, 1950.

[13] Parisini P, Di Silvestre M, Greggi T, Miglietta A, Paderni S. Lumbar disc excision in children and adolescents. Spine;26:1997–2000, 2001.

[14] Lee CX, Ranching W, Glenn W. Lateral lumbar spinal canal stenosis. Classification, pathology anatomy and surgical decompression. Spine;13:313–320, 1980.

[15] Haward S, Glover MJ. Lumbar spinal stenosis: historical perspectives, classification, and pathoanatomy. Semin Spine Surg;6(2):69–77, 1994.

[16] Thomas SA. Spinal stenosis: history and physical examination. Phys Med Rehabil Clin N Am;14:29–39, 2003.

[17] Inoue Nozomu MD, Orias AE. Biomechanics of interverebral disc degeneration. Orthop Clin North Am;42(4):487–499, 2011.

[18] Kirkaldy-Willis WH, Farfan HF. Instability of the lumbar spine. Clin Orthop Relat Res. 1982 May;(165):110-23.

[19] Deyo RA, Gray DT, Kreuter W et al. United States trends in lumbar fusion surgery for degenerative conditions. Spine;30:1441–1445, 2005.

[20] Epstein NE, Maldonado VC, Cusik JF. Symptomatic lumbar spinal stenosis. Surg Neurol;50:3–10, 1998.

[21] Arnoldi CC, Brodsky AE, Cauchoix J et al. Lumbar spinal stenosis and nerve root entrapment: syndromes, definition and classification. Clin Orthop;115:4–5, 1976.

[22] Hall S, Bartleson JD, Onoforio BM et al. Lumbar spinal stenosis. Clinical features, diagnostic procedures and results of surgical treatment in 68 patients. Ann Intern Med; 103(2):271–275, 1985.

[23] Naylor A. Factors in the development of the spina stenosis syndrome. J Bone Joint Surg Br;61(3):319–328, 1978

[24] Blau JN, Logue V. Intermittent claudication of the cauda equina. Lancet;1:1081–1086, 1961.

[25] Johnsson KE, Rosen I, Uden A. The natural course of lumbar spinal stenosis. Clin Orthop;279:82–86, 1992.

[26] Dyck P, Doyle JB. Bicycle test of Van Gelderen in diagnosis of intermittent cauda equina compression syndrome. J Neurosurg;46:667–670, 1997.

[27] Denn HG, Zimmerman RS, Lyons MK et al. Measurement of exercise tolerance on the treadmill test in patients with symptomatic lumbar spinal stenosis: a useful indicator of functional status and surgical outcome. J Neurosurg;83:27–30, 1995.

[28] Fritz JM, Erhard RE, Delitto A et al. Preliminary results of the two-stage treadmill test as a clinical diagnostic tool in the differential diagnosis of the lumbar spinal stenosis. J Spinal Disord;10:410–416, 1997.

[29] Olszewski AD, Yaszemski MJ, White AA III. The anatomy of the human lumbar ligamentum flavum: new observations and their surgical importance. Spine;21:2307–2312, 1996.

[30] Sairyo K, Biyani A, Goel V et al. Pathomechanism of ligamentum flavum hypertrophy: a multidisciplinary investigation based on clinical, biomechanical, histologic, and biologic assessments. Spine;23:2649–2656, 2005.

[31] Katz JN, Dagas M, Stucki G et al. Degenerative lumbar spinal stenosis: diagnostic value of the history and physical examination. Arthrit Rheum;38(9):1236–1241, 1995.

[32] Spengler DM. Current concepts review. Degenerative stenosis of the lumbar spine. J Bone Joint Surg;69-A:305–308, 1987.

[33] Dyck P, Doyle JP Jr. "Bicycle Test" of Van Gelderen in diagnosis of intermittent cauda equina compression syndrome. Case Report/Neurosurgery;46:667–670, 1977.

[34] Arnoldi CC, Brodsky AE, Cauchoix J, et al. Lumbar spinal stenosis and nerve root entrapment syndromes. Definition and classification. Clin Orthop Relat Res. 1976 Mar-Apr;(115):4–5.

[35] Frymoyer JW, Newberg A, Pope MH, Wilder DG, Clements J, Macpherson B. Spine radiographs in patients with low-back pain. An epidemiological study in men. J Bone Joint Surg Am;66(7):1048–1055, 1984.

[36] Herkowitz HN, Garfin SR, Bell GR, Bumphrey F, Rothman RH. The use of computerized tomography in evaluating non-visualized vertebral levels caudad to a complete block on a lumbar myelogram. A review of thirty-two cases. J Bone Joint Surg Am;69(2): 218–224, 1987.

[37] Czervionke LF. Lumbar intervertebral disc disease. Neuroimaging Clin N Am;3:465–485, 1993.

[38] Hamanishi C, Matukura N, Fujita M, Tomihara M, Tanaka S. Crosssectional area of the stenotic lumbar dural tube measured from the transverse views of MRI. J Spinal Dis; 7:388–393, 1994.

[39] Owlia MB, Salimzadeh A, Alishiri G, Haghighi A. Comparison of two doses of corticosteroid in epidural steroid injection for lumbar radicular pain. Singapore Med J; 48(3):241–245, 2007.

[40] Amundsen T, Weber H, NOrdal HJ, Magnaes B et al. Lumbar spinal stenosis: conservative or surgical management? A prospective 10 year study. Spine;25(11):1424–1435, 2000.

[41] Haig AJ, Tong HC, Yamakawa KS, Quint DJ et al. The sensitivity and specificity of eletrodiagnostic testing for the clinical syndrome of lumbar stenosis. Spine;30(23): 2667–2676, 2005.

[42] Atlas SJ, Kelle RB, Wu YA et al. Long-term outcomes of surgical and nonsurgical management of lumbar spinal stenosis: 8 to 10 years results from the Maine Lumbar Spine Study. Spine;30(8):936–943, 2005.

[43] Waters WC, Bono CM, Gilbert TJ et al. An evidence based clinical guideline for the diagnosis and treatment of degenerative lumbar spondylolisthesies. Spine J;8(2):305–310, 2008.

[44] Chou R, Qasemm A, Snow V et al. Diagnosis and treatment of low back pain: a joint clinical practice guideline from the American college of physicians and the American Pain Society. Ann Intern Med;147(7):478–491, 2007 Oct 2.

[45] Stephane G, Steven JA . Lumbar spinal stenosis. Best Pract Res Clin Rheumatol;24(2): 253–265, 2010 April.

[46] Yaksi A, Ozgonenel L, Ozgonenel B. The efficiency of gabapentin in patients with lumbar spinal stenosis. Spine;32(9):939–942, 2007.

[47] Rodrigues LC, Natour J. A double-blind, randomized controlled, prospective trial assessing the effectiveness of oral corticoids in the treatment of symptomatic lumbar canal stenosis. J Negat Results Bioemed;13:13, 2014.

[48] Rittemberg JD, Ross AE. Functional rehabilitation for degenerative lumbar spina stenosis. Phys Med Rehabil Clin N Am (14);111–120, 2003.

[49] Whtiman JM. Flyn TW, Frotz JM. Nonsurgical management of patients with lumbar spine stenosis: a literature review and a case series of three patients managed with physical therapy. Phys Med Rehabil Clin N Am;14(1):77–101, 2003.

[50] Whitman JM, Flym TW, Chids JD, Wainer RS et al. A comparassion between two physical therapy treatment programs for patients with lumbar spinal stenosis: a randomized clinical trial. Spine;31(2):2541–2549, 2006.

[51] Zarife K, Suheda O, Kncuy S et al. Effectiveness of physical therapy and epidural steroid injections in lumbar spinal stenosis. Spine;34(10):985–989, 2009.

[52] Parr AT, Diwan S, Adbdi S. Lumbar interlaminar epidural injections in managing chronic low back and lower extremity pain: a systematic review. Pain Physician;12(1): 163–188, 2009 Jan–Feb.

[53] Cosgrove JL, Berlote M, Chase SL et al. Epidural steroid injections in the treatement of lumbar spinal stenosis efficacy and predictability of successful response. Am J Phys Med Reabil;90:1050–1055, 2011.

[54] Charles DR, Neil K, Ralph B, Kathy V. A retrospective analysis of the efficacy of epidural steroid injections. Clin Orthopaed Relat Res;228;270–273, 1998.

[55] Cuckler JM, Bernini PA, Wiesel SW et al. The use of epidural steroids in the treatment of lumbar radicular pain. J Bone Joint Surg Am;67:63–66, 1995.

[56] Fukusaki M, Kobayashi I, Tetsuya H Sumikawa K. Symptoms of spinal stenosis do not improve after epidural steroid injection. Clin J Pain;14:148–151, 1988.

[57] Shabat S, Arizon Z, Folman Y et al. Long-term outcomes of decompressive surgery for lumbar spinal stenosis in octogenarians. Eur Spine J;17:193–198, 2008.

[58] Airaksinen O, Hermo A, Saari T. Surgical treatment of lumbar spinal stenosis: patients postoperative disability and working capacity. Eur Spine J;3;261–264, 1994.

[59] Hurri H, Slatis P, Soini J et al. Lumbar spinal stenosis: assemtment of long-term outcome 12 years after operative and conservative treatment. J Spinal Disord;11:110–115, 1998.

[60] Atlas SJ, Keller RB, Robson D et al. Surgical and nossurgical manangement of lumbar spinal stenosis: four-years outcomes from the Maine lumbar spine study. Spine;25:556–562, 2000.

[61] Atlas SJ, Keller RB, Wu YA et al. Long-term outcomes of surgical and nonsurgical management of lumbar spine study. Spine;30:936–943, 2005.

[62] Turner JA, Ersek M, Herron L, Deyo R. Surgery for spinal stenosis: attempt meta-analysis of the literature. Spine;17:1–8, 1992.

[63] Ra'kerry KR, Douglas DN, Daniel EG, Kornelis AP, Steven CL. Lumbar spinal stenosis. Curr Orthop Pract;19(4):351–356, 2008.

[64] Asgarzadie F, Khoo LT. Minimally invasive operative management for lumbar spinal stenosis: overview of early and long-term outcomes. Orthop Clin N Am;38:387–399, 2007.

[65] Zucherman JF, Hsu KY, Hartjen CA, et al. A prospective randomized multicenter study for the treatment of lumbar spinal stenosis with the X stop interspinous implant: 1-year results. Eur Spine J;13:22–31, 2004.

[66] Deburg A, Bex M, Lassale B, Bitan F. Technique chirurgicale dans le traitement des Stenoses du canal Lombaire. Acta Orthop Belg;53:412–419, 1987.

[67] Spinavak J. Degenerative lumbar spinal stenosis. J Bone Joint Surg (Am);80-A:1053–1066, 1998.

[68] Yamada K, Matsuda H, Nabeta M et al. Clinical outcomes of microscopic decompression for degenerative lumbar foraminal stenosis: a comparison between patients with and without degenerative lumbar scoliosis. Eur Spine J;20:947–953, 2011.

[69] Richards JC, Manjubar S, Lindsey DP. The treatment mechanism of an interspinous process implant for lumbar neurogenic intermittent claudication. Spine;30:744–749, 2005.

[70] Siddiqui M, Nicol M, Karadimas E et al. The positional magnetic resonance imaging changes in the lumbar spine following insertion of a novel interspinous process distraction device. Spine;30:2677–2682, 2005.

[71] Turner J, Ersek M, Herron L et al. Patient outcomes after lumbar spinal fussions. JAMA; 268:907–911, 1992.

[72] Fairbank J. Frost H, Macdonald W, Yu L et al. Randomised controled trial to compare surgical stabilization of the lumbar spine with an intensive rehabilitation programme for patients with chronico low back pain: the MRC spine stabilization trial. Br Med J. 2005 May 28;1–7 330(7502): 1233.

[73] Herkowitz HN, Garfin SR. Indications and surgical results of arthrodesis following spinal stenosis Spinal Stenosis. Philadelphia: Ed. Sauders. The Spine 1999;p. 806M-T. 132.

[74] Fredmann B, Arizon Z, Zohar E et al. Observations on the safety and efficacy of surgical decompression for lumbar spinal stenosis in geriatric patients. Eur Spine J;11:571–574, 2002.

[75] Jolles BM, Porchet F, Theumann N. Surgical treatment of lumbar spinal stenosis. J Bone Joint Surg (Br);83:949–953, 2001.

[76] Alto TJ, Mallmivaara A, Kovacs F et al. Preoperative predictors for postoperative clinical outcome in lumbar spinal stenosis: systematic review. Spine;31(18):E648–E663, 2006.

[77] Genevay S, Atlas SJ. Lumbar spinal stenosis. Best Pract Res Clin Rheumatol;24(2);253–265, 2010.

[78] Eismont FJ, Wiesel SW, Rothman RH. Treatment of dural tears associated with spinal surgery. J Bone Joint Surg Am;63:1132–1136, 1981.

[79] Sin AH, Caldito G, Smith D et al. Predictive factors for dural tear and cerebrospinal leakage in patients undergoing lumbar surgery. J Neurosurg Spine;5:224–227, 2006.

Chapter 6

Surgical Treatment of Spinal Meningiomas

Antonino Raco, Alessandro Pesce and
Massimo Miscusi

Additional information is available at the end of the chapter

http://dx.doi.org/10.5772/64421

Abstract

Spinal meningiomas are common spinal tumors; in most cases they are benign and with a good surgical prognosis. However, specific location, infiltration of spinal cord, vascular encasement, or spinal root involvement can bring to a less favorable prognosis. We reviewed a series of 173 consecutive patients with spinal meningiomas treated from 1976 to 2011 in our institution, and data were stratified according to sex, age, symptoms, axial location, Simpson resection grade, and functional pre-/postoperative status. Particular attention was paid to description of those factors leading to a poor outcome. Functional improvement at follow-up was observed in 86.7% of cases, 6.4% of patients resulted stable, and 6.9% worsened; a low functional grade before surgery was connected to a lesser improvement after. Anterolateral meningiomas were the most represented (42.2%); a gross total resection (Simpson grade I and II) was conducted in 98.8% and a macroscopically complete removal without dural resection or coagulation (Simpson grade III) was performed in 1.2%. According to data from our series, negative prognostic factors seem to be: anterior or anterolateral axial implant, long-lasting symptoms before diagnosis, WHO grade > I, Simpson grade II and III resection, sphincter involvement, and worse functional grade at onset.

Keywords: spinal meningiomas, surgery, spinal tumors, recurrence, surgical outcome

1. Introduction

Spinal meningiomas (SM) account for 1.2–12% of CNS meningiomas, being relatively uncommon [1–3]. The typical clinical presentation consists of pain [4], followed by gait, sensory, and sphincter disturbances. The constant improvement of neuroimaging techniques, the use of intraoperative neuromonitoring, and the increasing reliability of the contemporary surgical tools have further improved the prognosis of SM, already recognized as excellent by Cushing and Eisenhardt [5], more than 80 years ago, in their historical monograph. Since this cornerstone in SM literature, many series confirmed this finding [1, 6–9]. However, cases of anteriorly located or calcified lesions, cases of recurrences, and cases in which there is violation of the arachnoidal layer, invasion of spinal cord parenchyma, and encasement of vascular structure stand as exceptions to this rule.

2. Incidence, location, and subtypes

SM count for 25–46% of the intradural-extramedullary lesions, second to spinal schwannomas, which is the most frequent entity of this location [10]. SM favor females [4, 6, 11, 12], its incidence is significantly higher in Caucasians and Asian Pacific islanders than in Afro-Americans and Native Americans [13].

Despite being described at every age [14, 15], the highest incidence is in the fifth and sixth decade age group [4, 6, 7, 11]. Below the age of 18, predilection for female sex is not present. This feature, matched with a peak of incidence during peri-menopausal period, is consistent with the widely described and recognized neoplastic cells responsitivity to female sex hormones, similar to what happens for intracranial meningiomas [11, 12]. The exact incidence of SM is not known even though is estimated about 0.5–2 cases per 100,000 persons per year [3].

The relatively higher incidence in the thoracic spine is also noted in current literature compared to the other biomechanically active segments [6–8, 16]. The dural attachment is most frequently found in the anterior/anterolateral dura. Our series (**Figure 1** and **Table 1**) confirms these data [1, 2, 6, 7].

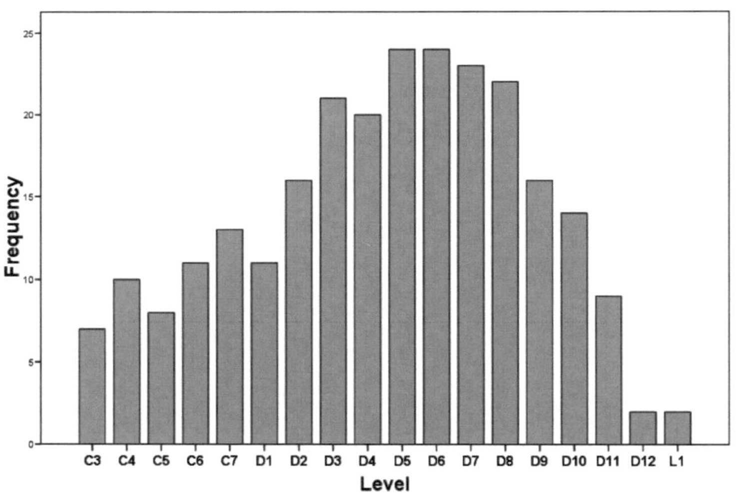

Figure 1. Incidence of spinal meningiomas in our cohort according to sagittal topography.

http://dx.doi.org/10.5772/64421

Total no. of patients	224
Lost to follow-up	15
Incomplete report (clinical and surgical)	22
Lesion involving CVJ	14
Residual cohort	173
Sex	
Woman	138 (79.8%)
Men	35 (20.2%)
Age	55.6 ± 13.1 years
Clinical presentation	
Pain	57 (32.9%)
Motor or gait disorders	55 (31.8%)
Paresthesias	53 (30.6%)
Sensory deficit	8 (4.6%)
Mean duration of preoperative symptoms	20.01 ± 18.86 months (range, 0–120 months)
Axial topography	
Posterior	11 (6.4%)
Posterolateral	42 (24.3%)
Anterolateral	73 (42.2%)
Anterior	15 (8.7%)
Lateral	32 (18.5%)
Simpson grade of resection	
I	52 pts (30%)
II	119 pts (68.8%)
III	2 pts (1.2%)
Neurological status at follow-up	
Improved	150 (86.7%)
Stable	11 (6.4%)
Worsened	12 (6.9%)
Sagittal topography according to biomechanical levels of the spine	
Subaxial cervical	14.2%
Cervicothoracic Junction	9.5%
Thoracic spine	75.5%
Thoracolumbar Junction	0.8%
Complications	
Total complication rate	7 (4.04%)
CSF leakage	3 (1.73%)
Spinal epidural hematoma	2 (1.15%)
Syringomyelia	1 (0.58%)
Adverse reaction to dural sealant	1 (0.58%)
WHO grading of the lesions	
I	170 pts (98.3%)
II	2 pts (1.15%)
III	1 pt (0.58%)

Table 1. Details of the final cohort.

SM histological subtypes are the same as their intracranial counterpart. The percentage of atypical/anaplastic SM is significantly lower than intracranial meningiomas [12]. In our series, WHO Grade I (**Table 1**) was the most represented subgroup of lesions in our cohort (98.3% of the lesions). These data are similar to other series [4, 6, 11, 12].

A higher incidence of SM is also well documented in patients suffering from neurofibromatosis. When a SM is detected in early life, it should raise suspicion of neurofibromatosis, especially in patients below the fourth decade and with extrathoracic sagittal location [12].

3. Diagnosis

3.1. Symptoms and physical findings

Literature recognize pain as the typical symptom at clinical onset of SM [6, 7, 17]. Pain can be axial, radicural, or radiating to upper or lower limbs, depending on the location of the tumor; it is commonly associated with paresthesias, hot and cold sensations, and sensory disturbances, followed by gait instability evolving in an obvious motor deficit, which is usually late due to the typical growth slowness of this lesions [2]. Sphincter impairment is a late finding and involves from 15 to 40% of the patients [18].

In our cohort, the most common disturbance at clinical onset was pain in 32.9% of cases (57 patients), followed by motor and gait disorder in 31.8% of cases, (55 patients); less frequently we observed paresthesias (30.6%, 53 patients), and occasionally a pure sensory disturbance was detectable (4.6%, 8 patients). Only 18.5% of patients complained a single disturbance at onset. The second disturbance in order of appearance was a motor disorder (61 patients, 35.3%) and occasionally a sphincter disturbance (10 patients, 5.8%). The average duration of symptoms was 20.01±18.86 months (range, 0–120 months) (**Table 1**).

Pain was described as axial (cervical or thoracic; 30 patients; 17.34%), radicular (radiating to corresponding dermatome; 5 patients; 2.89%), or radiating to distant dermatomes (e.g. thoracic cord meningiomas with pain radiating to lower limbs; 22 patients; 12.71%). A total of 21 patients (12.13%) were retrospectively estimated to suffer from a pure radiculopathy, 37 from a pure myelopathy (21.38%), and 115 from myeloradiculopathy (66.47%).

3.2. Radiology

Standard X-ray plain film is of limited value, it may demonstrate pedicle or soma erosion, abnormalities in the normal spine curvatures [18]. X-ray standard myelography may outline a contrast block at the level of the extradural lesion, but it has been disused in the common everyday clinical practice. Spine contrast-enhanced CT scans provide detailed information about bony anatomy; it finds a contemporary huge value while investigating extensively calcified lesions or in defining the detailed anatomy of recurrent SM [6, 17].

Since its introduction (at our Institution in 1991), a preoperative magnetic resonance imaging (MRI) scans have become the gold standard in defining this pathology. T1w, T2w, T1w

http://dx.doi.org/10.5772/64421

gadolinium-enhanced sequences are routinely performed to investigate anatomical details of the lesions (**Figure 2A, B, E,** and **F**). Gadolinium-enhanced MRI imaging demonstrated an homogeneously enhanced mass delocating spinal cord parenchyma and nerve roots, intra-extradural extension of the lesion, and dural tail; it may not sufficiently help the differential diagnosis between spinal schwannomas and meningiomas [14].

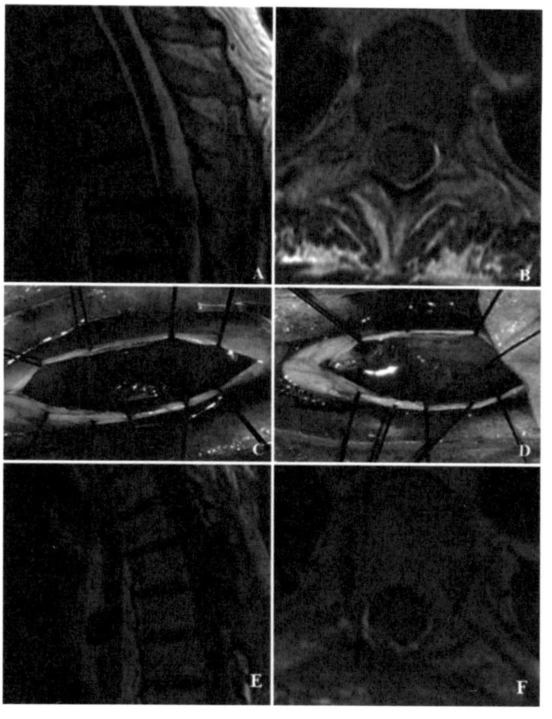

Figure 2. A. Sagittal T2w and B. Axial T1w gadolinium enhanced images of a thoracic spinal meningioma causing spinal cord dislocation. C. Intraoperative pre- and D. post- total resection of the lesion. Dura mater was extensively coagulated with no remnant of the disease, realizing a Simpson Grade of Resection II. E. Sagittal and F. Axial T1w gadolinium enhanced postoperative MRI demonstrating complete resection of the tumor and spinal cord decompression.

4. Surgical treatment—technical standards, pitfalls, and advances

Standard prone position is commonly used to approach a SM. Mayfield clamp may prove useful in cases of high subaxial cervical SM. A preoperative radioscopic localization of the involved levels is routinely carried out. After a standard midline skin incision and hypodermal tissues sharp dissection, fascia is incised in a standard midline fashion, and subperiostal exposure of laminae and articular processes is performed. A standard laminotomy (or hemilaminectomy) exposes the dural sac. In case of thoracic spine anterior/anterolateral axially located lesion, a costo-trasversectomy to enlarge surgical corridor can be performed. Midline temporary 4 or 5-0 silk tack-up sutures lead to a safer midline dural opening. Under magnification of the operative microscope, a microsurgical lesionectomy is performed (**Figure 2C** and **D**). Regardless of the potential infiltrative pattern or encasement of spinal vascular structures and nerve roots, a CUSA debulking is made to avoid any traction on the spinal cord.

Total removal is the target in all posteriorly located lesions, dural attachment must be removed, and a duraplasty completes the procedure. For anterior/anterolateral lesions, macroscopically complete excision is always associated with generous coagulation of the dural attachment.

Experience and literature have led us to strongly prefer laminotomy over laminectomy to perform a standard posterior midline approach for the evidence-based risk of iatrogenic postoperative instability. In order to clarify the difference between laminectomy and laminotomy, we use the term "laminotomy" to describe a "partial laminectomy" sparing of the medial facet of the articular process.

The reported incidence of postoperative instability in cervical spine is as high as 56% in more than four-level laminectomies and 11% in less than four level [19], whereas in thoracolumbar spine, instability appears in 25% of patients receiving more than two-level laminectomies [20]. Postoperative deformity is reported in 9.4% of patients receiving laminectomy compared to 3% of patients receiving laminotomy [21].

In most cases, a standard posterior approach allows surgeon to work in an adequate surgical corridor to achieve complete excision even for anterior/anterolateral lesions. In our experience, standard posterior approach is the gold standard in huge number of cases. However, intraextradural lesion with infiltration of the vertebral body, massively calcified lesions, anterior/anterolateral lesions, or recurrent tumors with spinal cord invasion stand as notable exceptions to this rule. In these cases, lateral or anterior approaches, with generous arthrectomy, pedicle resection, and partial/total vertebrectomy, performed to gain an optimal attachment control and safer spinal cord manipulation may be required [8, 16, 22, 23].

5. Neurological and functional outcome and complications

SM are slowly growing lesion, typically benign. Usually, they carry a fair neurological and functional prognosis [1, 6–9]. However, cases of anteriorly located or calcified lesions, recurrences, and cases in which there is violation of the arachnoidal layer, invasion of spinal cord parenchyma, and encasement of vascular structure stand as exceptions to this rule.

For this reason, one of the major efforts in SM surgery research and literature has historically been to preoperatively identify cases with a worse functional and neurological prognosis.

With the same aforementioned purpose, we critically reviewed our entire cohort of patients operated on for SM excision through a detailed retrospective analysis. Functional and neurological data about the outcome of each patient were recoded with Frankel [24] and McCormick [25] scales.

Frankel scale is a functional evaluation scale, initially conceived for spinal cord injury (SCI) but capable of assessing residual function "below" the level of a lesion. It is extremely easy and extremely sensitive with respect to coarse variations of the spinal cord function. McCormick scale, designed for intramedullary neoplasms, provides information about spinal cord function in relation to the quality of life and patient's independence (e.g. walking ability and the degree of impairment in the upper limbs). In our cohort, these scales appear to be strongly associated (Pearson's bivariate correlation p 0.01; r= −0.820 McCormick Pre-Frankel, Frankel −0.934 McCormick at Follow-Up), validating each other.

The scales are reported in **Table 2**.

	Frankel scale
A	Complete neurological injury—no motor or sensory function below the level of the injury
B	Preserved sensation only—no motor function below the level of the injury
C	Preserved motor nonfunctional—some motor function observed below the level of the injury
D	Preserved motor function—useful motor function below the level of the injury
E	Normal motor—no clinically detected abnormality in motor or sensory function with normal sphincter function; abnormal reflexes and subjective sensory abnormalities may be present
	McCormick scale
1	Intact neurologically, normal ambulation, and minimal dysesthesia
2	Mild motor or sensory deficit and functional independence
3	Moderate deficit, limitation of function, and independent w/external aid
4	Severe motor or sensory deficit, limited function, and dependent
5	Paraplegia or quadriplegia, even w/flickering movement

Table 2. Frankel and McCormick scales.

The preoperative Frankel functional classes most represented in our cohort were classes A, B, and C (respectively 15, 9, and 91 patients, amounting to 66.5% of the total). These classes reflect a deeper neurological impairment. Preoperative McCormick grade III, IV, and V was recorded, respectively, in 76, 36, and 18 patients (75.1% of the sample), whereas in the postoperative period, A, B, and C and III, IV, and IV classes were represented by 28.3% (49 patients) and 28.6% (53 patients).

The number of patients who experienced a significant improvement at follow-up amounted to 150 (86.7%), 11 were stable (6.4%) and the remaining 12 worsened (6.9%). In this cohort, the worst functional preoperative status showed a clear tendency to more modest improvements both on Frankel and McCormick scales (Pearson's bivariate correlation, both p 0.01, r = 0.511 and 0.618).

In our sample, a long duration of preoperative symptoms and severe preoperative impairment are related to worse outcomes; this result is similar to other reports [8, 26]. The author (A.R.) has previously reported a clear possibility of recovery even in patients harboring deep functional preoperative impairment [26], outlining that age (under 60) and duration of preoperative impairment stand as the most important predictors of neurological recovery.

Anteriorly located lesions imply the most difficult setting in SM surgery [4, 7, 8, 12]. Consistent with the literature [7, 8], in our series, anterior/anterolateral lesions were identified as a subgroup with worse outcome compared to different axial topographies. Purely anterior lesions with arachnoidal adhesions to spinal cord and vascular encasement lead to an increased risk of spinal cord traction and surgical damage.

Some authors report massive calcification of the lesion as a predictor of neurological postoperative deterioration [6, 8]. In our series, only three patients harbored massively calcified spinal meningiomas, and thus this feature failed to reach statistical significance to confirm these findings.

Recurrence of SM in our sample was predictive of worse outcome. Our recurrence rate was 2.3% (4/173 cases). In the current literature, this rate varies between 1.3 and 13% [2, 4, 6, 9, 14, 18, 27, 28]. Obviously, WHO grading of the lesions is correlated with the probability of local relapses. In recurrent SM surgery, arachnoidal scarring caused by the first procedure can make tumor debulking harder and, despite the regular use of intraoperative neuromonitoring and CUSA, can lead to a worse outcome. In our cohort, patients harboring recurrent lesions were 4, a total of just two patients underwent a second SM excision surgery, and, although under-represented compared to the entire sample (2 of 4 patients on 173 patients of the entire cohort), showed a statistical association with worse outcomes. Therefore, whenever feasible, our experience suggests, according to Literature, that first surgery should always be as aggressive as possible [7, 23].

No postoperative death was recorded in our sample. Mortality rate in SM surgery is usually extremely low, ranging between 0.8 and 2% in series reported after 1999 [6–8].

6. Complications

In SM surgery, complications can be coarsely divided in two subgroups: neurological postoperative worsening and surgical complications causing neurological impairment. Among the last subgroup, most common surgical complications include spinal epidural hematoma, CSF leakage with or without deep or superficial infections, syringomyelia, and iatrogenic instability [2, 6, 7, 19–21].

The first subgroup was extensively discussed in the previous paragraph as well as concerns about iatrogenic instability are described in surgical treatment section.

Surgical complications counted for a total of 7/173 cases (4.04% of patients). A total of four patients (two postoperative spinal epidural hematoma, one syringomyelia, and one adverse reaction to dural sealant) required a revision surgery. The remaining underwent conservative treatments (three patients with CSF leakage resolved with lumbar drainage).

Lumbar drainage is reserved for the management of at least 4–5 days of persistent wound CSF leakage. In this series, three patients suffered from wound CSF leakage and were treated conservatively by bedrest and lumbar drainage positioning. These complications were completely resolved in 5–7 days and did not require a surgical revision. Lumbar drainage use for CSF leakages treatment is hugely validated by experience and literature [29, 30].

No case of deep or superficial infection was recorded in our series. According to contemporary Literature, at present, deep and superficial infections are exceptional complications [7, 17].

7. Simpson grade of resection and recurrences

In the spinal compartment, recurring lesions are less common than meningiomas rising within the intracranial compartment (10–26%) [4]. Mirimanoff et al. [28] showed that the long-term follow-up of patients operated on for spinal meningioma removal can indicate up to 13% of recurrence at 10 years. However, the main limitation of this study is the small size of the cohort investigated (18 patients). Nakamura et al. [23] reported a recurrence rate as high as 30% at 12-year follow-up for patients who received a Simpson grade II resection. Setzer et al. [16] reported a stratification of recurrence probability by WHO histological grading: 1.4% for grade I, 50% for grade II, and 100% for grade III and IV, in 43.5 ± 24.8 months of follow-up.

As previously mentioned, recurrence of SM in our sample was predictive of worse outcome. Our recurrence rate was 2.3% (4/173 cases). In the current literature, this rate varies between 1.3 and 13% [2, 4, 6, 9, 14, 18, 27, 28].

Simpson grade I was obtained in 52 patients (30%). In all these cases, dural attachment, mainly posterior or posterolateral, was removed and a duraplasty with eterologous dural patch was performed. The rationale for this procedure is that literature analysis reveals a difference in terms of recurrence probability for Simpson grade I and II [2, 18, 23], and these data are confirmed in our series. In case of duraplasty, dural sealant was routinely used, since its use is substantially supported by literature [31].

Our routine postoperative SM follow-up protocol consists of a minimum 4 years of clinical and radiological follow-up reserved for patients with Simpson grade of resection I and WHO grade I lesions. Simpson grade of resection > I and WHO grade > I patients underwent a closer clinical and radiological follow-up. Such a follow-up protocol appears justified in relation to the natural history of SM, an extremely slowly growing lesion, which favors fifth/sixth decade. Some recurrences may be ignored because they never reach clinical significance in the lifespan of the patient. Our policy toward recurrent lesions is to reoperate only on those with MRI-demonstrated progressive regrowth tendency, because, according to literature and experience, operating a recurrent SM is often technically challenging [7, 8, 32, 33].

8. Conclusions

Spinal meningiomas are common primary spinal tumors, in most cases benign and with a good surgical prognosis. However, specific location, infiltration of spinal cord, vascular encasement, or spinal root involvement can bring on to a less favorable prognosis. We can adfirm that the negative prognostic factors in our study were: anterior or anterolateral axial location, protracted symptoms before diagnosis, WHO Grade > I, Simpson grade II and III resection, sphincter involvement, and worse functional grade at onset.

Author details

Antonino Raco[1], Alessandro Pesce[1*] and Massimo Miscusi[2]

*Address all correspondence to: ale_pesce83@yahoo.it

1 "Sapienza" University, Rome, Italy

2 "ICOT" Hospital, Latina – "Sapienza" Univesity, Rome, Italy

References

[1] Bret P, Lecuire J, Lapras C, Deruty R, Dechaume JP, Assaad A. Intraspinal meningiomas. A series of 60 cases. Neurochirurgie. 1976; 22:5–22.

[2] Solero CL, Fornari M, Giombini S, Lasio G, Oliveri G, Cimino C, Pluchino F. Spinal meningiomas: review of 174 operated cases. Neurosurgery. 1989; 25:153–160.

[3] Westwick HJ, Shamji MF. Effects of sex on the incidence and prognosis of spinal meningiomas: a Surveillance, Epidemiology, and End Results study. J Neurosurg Spine. 2015; 29:1-6.

[4] Maiuri F, De Caro ML, de Divitiis O, Vergara P, Mariniello G. Spinal meningiomas: Age-related features, Clin Neurol Neurosurg. 2011; 113(1):34–38.

[5] Cushing H, Eisenhardt L. Meningiomas: Their Classification, Regional Behavior, Life History, and Surgical End Results. Springfield, IL, Charles C Thomas, 1938.

[6] Sandalcioglu EI, Hunold A, Muller O, Bassiouni H, Stolke D, Asgari S. Spinal meningiomas: Critical review of 131 surgically treated patients. Eur Spine J. 2008; 17:1035–1041.

[7] Klekamp J, Samii M. Surgical results for spinal meningiomas. Surg Neurol.1999; 52(6): 552–562.

[8] Westwick HJ, Yuh SJ, Shamji MF. Complication avoidance in the resection of spinal meningiomas. World Neurosurg. 2015; 83(4):627-634.

[9] Roux FX, Nataf F, Pinaudeau M, Borne G, Devaux B, Meder JF. Intraspinal meningiomas: review of 54 cases with discussion of poor prognosis factors and modern therapeutic management. Surg Neurol. 1996; 46(5):458–463.

[10] Albanese V, Platania N. Spinal intradural extramedullary tumors. J Neurosurg Sci. 2002; 16:18–24.

[11] Yoon SH, Chung CK, Jahng TA. Surgical outcome of spinal canal meningiomas, J Kor Neurosurg Soc. 2007; 42(4):300-304.

[12] Saracenia C, Harropb J. Spinal meningioma: Chronicles of contemporary neurosurgical diagnosis and management. Clin Neurol Neurosurg. 2009; 111(3):221–226.

[13] Kshettry VR, Hsieh JK, Ostrom QT, Kruchko C, Benzel EC, Barnholtz-Sloan JS. Descriptive epidemiology of spinal meningiomas in the United States. Spine (Phila Pa 1976). 2015; 40(15):E886-E889.

[14] Cohen-Gadol AA, Zikel OM, Koch CA, Scheithauer BW, Krauss WE. Spinal meningiomas in patients younger than 50 years of age: a 21-year experience. J Neurosurg. 2003; 98(3 Suppl):258–263.

[15] Fortuna A, Nolletti A, Nardi P, Caruso R. Spinal neurinomas and meningiomas in children. Acta Neurochir (Wien). 1981. 55(3-4), 329-341.

[16] Setzer M, Vatter H, Marquardt G, Seifert V, Vrionis FD. Management of spinal meningiomas: surgical results and a review of the literature. Neurosurg Focus. 2007; 23(4):E14.

[17] Kleklamp J, Samii M. "Extramedullary Tumors" in Surgery of Spinal Tumors. 1st ed. Springer-Verlag Berlin Heidelberg. 2007. p. 248-260.

[18] Levy WJ Jr, Bay J, Dohn D. Spinal cord meningioma. J Neurosurg. 1982; 57(6):804–812

[19] Katsumi Y, Honma T, Nakamura T: Analysis of cervical instability resulting from laminectomies for removal of spinal cord tumor. Spine (Phila Pa 1976). 1989; 14(11): 1171-1176.

[20] Papagelopoulos PJ, Peterson HA, Ebersold MJ, Emmanuel PR, Choudhury SN, Quast LM. Spinal column deformity and instability after lumbar or thoracolumbar laminectomy for intraspinal tumors in children and young adults. Spine (Phila Pa 1976). 1997; 22(4):442-451.

[21] McGirt MJ, Garces-Ambrossi GL, Parker SL, et al. Short-term progressive spinal deformity following laminoplasty versus laminectomy for resection of intradural spinal tumors: analysis of 238 patients. Neurosurgery. 2010; 66(5):1005-1012.

[22] Arima H, Takami T, Yamagata T, et al. Surgical management of spinal meningiomas: A retrospective case analysis based on preoperative surgical grade. Surg Neurol Int. 2014; 5(Suppl 7): S333–S338.

[23] Nakamura M, Tsuji O, Fujiyoshi K, et al. Long-term surgical outcomes of spinal meningiomas. Spine (Phila Pa 1976). 2012; 37(10):E617-E623.

[24] Frankel HL, Hancock DO, Hyslop G, et al. The value of postural reduction in the initial management of closed injuries of the spine with paraplegia and tetraplegia. Paraplegia. 1969; 7(3):179-192.

[25] McCormick PC, Stein BM: Intramedullary tumors in adults. Neurosurg Clin N Am. 1990;1(3):609-630.

[26] Ciappetta P, Domenicucci M, Raco A. Spinal meningiomas: prognosis and recovery factors in 22 cases with severe motor deficits. Acta Neurol Scand. 1988; 77(1):27-30.

[27] Schick U, Marquaedt G, Lorenz R. Recurrence of benign spinal neoplasm. Neurosurg Rev. 2001; 24(1):20-25.

[28] Mirimanoff RO, Dosoretz DE, Linggood RM, Ojemann RG, Martuza RL. Meningioma: analysis of recurrence and progression following neurosurgical resection. J Neurosurg 1985; 62:18–24.

[29] Khan M. Rihn J, Steele G. et al. Postoperative management protocol for incidental dural tears during degenerative lumbar spine surgery: A review of 3,183 consecutive degenerative lumbar cases. Spine (Phila Pa 1976). 2006; 31(22): 2609-2613

[30] Shapiro SA, Scully T. Closed continuous drainage of cerebrospinal fluid via a lumbar subarachnoid catheter for treatment or prevention of cranial/spinal cerebrospinal fluid fistula. Neurosurgery 1992; 30(2):241-245.

[31] Weinstein JS, Liu KC, Delashaw JB Jr, et al. The safety and effectiveness of a dural sealant system for use with nonautologous duraplasty materials. J Neurosurg. 2010;112(2):428-433

[32] Caroli E, Acqui M, Roperto R, Ferrante L, D'Andrea G. Spinal en plaque meningiomas: a contemporary experience. Neurosurgery 2004; 55:1275–1279.

[33] Gezen F, Kahraman S, Canakci Z, Beduk A. Review of 36 cases of spinal cord meningioma. Spine (Phila Pa 1976). 2000; 25:727-731.

Chapter 7

Biomarkers of Acute Brain Injury in the Emergency Department

Linda Papa and Kimberly Rosenthal

Additional information is available at the end of the chapter

http://dx.doi.org/10.5772/64222

Abstract

The diagnosis of acute brain injury in the acute care setting is based on neurological examination and neuroimaging tools such as computed tomography (CT) scanning and magnetic resonance imaging (MRI). However, there are limitations to both CT and MRI scanning. The lack of objective, noninvasive and readily accessible clinical tools to detect injury has left clinicians with uncertainty about how to best identify and treat these conditions. It is also very difficult for patients and their families who struggle to better understand the deficits they deal with on a daily basis. There have been many studies exploring many promising biomarkers during the last decade. Despite the large number of published studies there is still a lack of any Food and Drug Administration (FDA)-approved biomarkers for brain injury in adults and children. Given all of these researches, there is now an important need to validate and introduce them into the clinical setting. This chapter reviews commonly studied biomarkers for acute brain injury in humans, with an emphasis on traumatic brain injury and stroke.

Keywords: biomarkers, acute, brain injury, traumatic brain injury, stroke, ischemic stroke, hemorrhagic stroke, subarachnoid hemorrhage, emergency department, neurosurgery, neuroimaging, neurosurgical intervention, migraine, diagnosis, prognosis, blood test, serum, cerebrospinal fluid, glial fibrillary acid protein, ubiquitin C-terminal hydrolase, S100B, tau, spectrin breakdown products, neurofilaments, neuron specific enolase, CT scan, magnetic resonance imaging (MRI)

1. Introduction

1.1. Epidemiology of acute neurological diseases and the evolution of acute brain injury biomarkers

Neurological biomarkers have considerable diagnostic and prognostic promise given their variety, range, and specificity, though despite the potential advantages of their use and the array of conditions to which they apply, biomarkers have yet to be broadly employed in the clinical setting [1–4]. Before assessing the roles of biomarkers in the diagnosis and prognosis of various acute neurological conditions, some consideration should first be given to the epidemiology of these conditions. Traumatic brain injury (TBI) results from external blunt force trauma to the head—most often through motor vehicle accidents, falls, and sports injuries—and is marked by cognitive and motor deficiency, the severity of which is determined via the Glasgow Coma Scale (GCS). TBI may be associated with bleeding (hematoma), brain swelling (cerebral edema), hydrocephalus, herniation, increased intracranial pressure, and microscopic damage to the neuronal and astrocyte network. An estimated 40% of acute injury deaths in the United States are attributed to TBI, with mortality rates highest among those aged 15–24 or 65 and older; individuals who are part of ethnic minority groups and possess lower socioeconomic status also suffer increased risk for TBI.

Stroke, comparatively, is characterized by a either an ischemic and a hemorrhagic insult and is both the third most common cause of mortality in the United States and, along with ischemic heart disease, the leading cause of mortality worldwide. Moreover, stroke is also the second leading cause of disability among the global population, with resulting complications ranging from vision impairments and aphasia to varying degrees of paralysis, short-term memory loss, dementia, and difficulty concentrating and learning novel information. Aneurysmal subarachnoid hemorrhage (SAH) is a degenerative sub-condition of stroke, inciting hydrocephalus, vasospasm, and continuous bleeding in 26–73% of patients. While the incidence of SAH in the United States ranged, as of 2010, from roughly 0.015 to 0.287% of the population, the mortality rate of SAH sufferers varies from 40 to 60%. Both age-controlled stroke incidence and subsequent medical and economic complications have especially intensified in both developing nations and lower-income communities. The symptomology and neuroimaging data of SAH in particular can often resemble that of acute migraine, for which it is mistaken in roughly 12–51% of diagnoses. Acute migraine afflicts approximately 18% of women and 6% of men in the United States. Despite the widespread prevalence of migraine and the significant physical and financial burden it poses to sufferers, the condition is often underdiagnosed.

In light of practitioners' concerns with timeliness, accuracy, and risk aversion in the diagnostic and treatment processes, serum biomarkers with reliable specificity for and sensitivity to various categories of brain injury are appetizing diagnostic and monitoring tools. This is especially so in contexts haunted by indeterminate, unavailable, or simply untimely neuroimaging, hence why biomarker panels would be of particular utility in more rural settings and non-hospital environments where rapid triage is especially critical. Although promising cerebrospinal fluid (CSF) biomarkers for hemorrhage, migraine, and stroke have been studied, serum biomarkers are needed. Having a blood test would eliminate the need for invasive procedures such as lumbar puncture, which tends to be a lengthy and physically uncomfortable process with potential complications. Biomarkers have also shown potential in evaluating injury severity such as brain infarction and in predicting post-stroke prognosis, thereby aiding health care workers in their assessment of the level of post-stroke care required by individual patients. It must be noted, however, that while both serum and CSF biomarkers are examined in the following chapter, the promptness with which serum samples can be collected and analyzed far exceeds that of CSF biomarkers; in addition, serum assays have the advantage of being able to be collected in the field or in settings where access to technical equipment is limited.

This chapter reviews some of the most widely studied biomarkers for acute brain injury in the clinical setting, with an emphasis on traumatic brain injury and stroke.

2. Biomarkers of astroglial injury

2.1. S100β

S100β is found in astrocytes and is a low-affinity calcium-binding protein [5] that helps to regulate intracellular levels of calcium. It is considered a marker of astrocyte injury or death. It can also be found in cells that are not neuronal such as adipocytes, chondrocytes, and melanoma cells, making it non-brain specific [6, 7]. S100β is one of the most extensively studied biomarkers for brain injury [2, 3, 8]. Elevated S100β levels in serum have been associated with increased incidence of post-concussive syndrome and problems with cognition and MRI abnormalities [9–13]. However, there are also a number of studies negating these findings [14–17]. Since many of these results have not been consistently reproduced, the clinical value of S100β in TBI, particularly mild TBI and concussion, is still controversial. A number of studies have found correlations between elevated serum levels of S100β and CT abnormalities in adults and children [3, 18]. Unfortunately, its utility in the setting of polytrauma remains controversial, because it is also elevated in trauma patients with peripheral trauma who had no direct head trauma [19–21].

S100B seems an equally suspect diagnostic tool for acute ischemic stroke. Several findings have placed peak S100B elevation at days 2–4 following acute ischemic stroke onset, rendering its measurement somewhat fruitless in the majority of ischemia cases in which recombinant tissue plasminogen activator (rt-PA) generally needs to be performed within the first three or, more rarely, 4.5 h, post-infarction onset. However, concerns with S100B's specificity are potentially less problematic when distinguishing hemorrhagic from ischemic stroke. Because morphological damage tends to be more immediate in cases of hemorrhaging than in ischemia, S100B concentrations have been shown to peak earlier in cases of hemorrhage, at roughly 24 h post-infarction onset. This timescale, however, might still be too prolonged to render S100B a viable diagnostic marker, although it should be noted that CAT scans are routinely given 24 h after ischemia onset in order to rule out hemorrhage. Moreover, research has tended to focus on the potential association between S100B and ischemia rather than hemorrhage.

Instead, S100B offers more promise as a prognostic tool in the evaluation of infarction severity in coordination with MRI results and, relatedly, patient outcome and functionality. S100B concentrations within the first 2–10 days after onset have been found to be predictive of infarct volume, potentially more so than NSE levels are, and moreover have correlated well with assessments of neurological functionality as measured by the National Institutes of Health Stroke Scale (NIHSS) [22]. The prognostic value of S100B is also exhibited in its potential to predict hemorrhagic transformation in patients who have suffered ischemia within 24 h. Moreover, Fassbender et al. found that ischemia resulting in legions greater than 5 cm in volume was correlated with significantly greater concentrations of S100B 10, 24, and 72 h post onset [22].

S100B has also been studied as a possible means by which to distinguish aneurysmal subarachnoid hemorrhage from acute migraine. Aneurysmal SAH is a degenerative condition, inciting continuous bleeding in 26–73% of patients [23, 24], as well as hydrocephalus and vasospasm [25]. It is not uncommon for SAH to be initially mistaken for migraine, especially since headache is a prominent symptom of both conditions, with the frequency of overall SAH misdiagnosis between 12 and 51% [26–30]. Indeed, physical symptoms of SAH and severe, acute-onset migraine are remarkably similar to one another. CT and MRI scans remain the most reliable means by which SAH can be diagnosed, the former more accurate in detection within the first 24 h following attack and the latter more accurate after 24 h have elapsed since attack onset. However, vasospasm can render imaging of the aneurysm through magnetic resonance angiography Magnetic resonance angiography (MRA) difficult. The error rate of such scans, especially due to their qualitative nature, may perhaps be improved upon by the use of diagnostic biomarkers. S100B concentrations have been shown to rise in response to acute migraine, peaking 2–4 days after onset during the "pain-free period," but detectable within 2–3 h of onset [31, 32]. Because S100B concentration time courses in SAH and migraine are similar, biomarkers such as NSE, which are characterized by more distinctive patterns in acute migraine, are likely more useful diagnostic tools.

2.2. Glial fibrillary acid protein (GFAP)

Glial fibrillary acidic protein (GFAP) is a protein found in astroglial skeleton and is found in both white and gray brain matter. It was first isolated by Eng et al. [33] and appears to be strongly upregulated during astrogliosis [34]. Serum GFAP has been shown to be elevated with various types of brain damage including neurodegenerative disorders [35, 36], stroke [37], and severe traumatic brain injury [19, 38–43]. In particular, GFAP has become a very promising brain-specific glial-derived biomarker for mild TBI in adults and children [14, 20, 21, 44–47]. GFAP is released into serum following a mild TBI within an hour of injury and remains elevated for several days after injury [21, 44, 47]. Unlike S100β, GFAP is elevated in mild TBI patients with axonal injury as evidenced by MRI at 3 months post injury [14]. In adults and children, serum GFAP levels distinguish mild TBI patients from trauma patients without TBI and detect intracranial lesions on CT with a sensitivity of 94–100% [20, 21, 44, 46, 47]. Moreover, GFAP outperforms S100β in detecting CT lesions in the setting of multiple trauma when extracranial fractures are present [21, 46]. GFAP also predicts the need for neurosurgical intervention in patients with mild TBI [44, 47]. The temporal profile of GFAP was evaluated in a large cohort of 584 trauma patients seen at the emergency department. GFAP performed consistently over 7 days in identifying concussion and mild to moderate TBI, detecting traumatic intracranial lesions on head computed tomography (CT), and predicting neurosurgical intervention [47].

GFAP promises to be an especially potent biomarker, perhaps providing the opportunity to reliably distinguishing ischemic and hemorrhagic stroke. The necessity of expeditiously distinguishing between the two subsets of stroke poses a particular difficulty because of the manner in and extent to which treatment paradigms vary between the stroke classes. While the securing of endovascular coils or surgical implantation of clips at the site of the aneurysm are viable treatment options for hemorrhage, rt-PA, a recombinant form of an endogenous serine protease used for thrombolysis, offers the only Food and Drug Administration (FDA)-approved treatment for ischemic stroke beyond supportive care. Studies have shown that the risk-benefit ratio of rt-PA administration is favorable for patients treated within 3 h of stroke onset, although some institutions place the threshold to 6 h [24, 48–51]. Mechanical thrombectomy, an endovascular procedure in which the offending clot is excised via stent retriever, is becoming an increasingly explored treatment method viable up to 6 h within the onset of stroke symptom presentation [52–54]. Even this treatment strategy for ischemic stroke, however, is not usually undertaken without having first administered rt-PA to the patient [55].

For both ischemic and hemorrhagic stroke, patient outcomes improve with more rapid treatment administration. Although swift use of rt-PA would benefit patients suffering from ischemic stroke, which comprises roughly 87% of stroke cases, clinical practitioners must be circumspect in their use of the treatment because of its detrimental effects on the 13% of individuals presenting with hemorrhagic stroke [56]. The administration of rt-PA in response to ischemic stroke, however, can only be as prompt as proper diagnosis. Healthcare providers are thus left with the difficult task of both rapidly confirming the diagnosis of stroke to ensure eligibility for treatment, and rapidly confirming that a patient is not at risk for significant hemorrhage [24, 48–51]. CT and MRI scans are currently the primary diagnostic means at a physician's disposal, though assessment also includes a focused medical history, physical exam, and blood work. However, CT scans are more readily available in most settings than MRI [25]. In some communities, portable CT scanners are available for use by emergency responders, though this particular technology is neither widely available nor cost-effective. MRI, in comparison, can be more sensitive than CT scans in determining the presence of both intracerebral hemorrhage and the degree of ischemia [26, 49]. However, recent studies have shown that even MRI scans can miss roughly 17% of strokes [28–30, 57, 58]. CT scans are even less effective. Studies indicate that less than half of patients with ischemic stroke will show characteristic changes on CT scan within 3 h of symptom onset [58]. Even more advanced imaging techniques such as perfusion-diffusion mismatch models have received criticism for their ability to accurately predict lesion growth. Hence, current imaging techniques, despite providing arguably our most reliable stroke diagnoses, may temporally limit the diagnosis of stroke and delay the provision of timely treatment. Stroke biomarkers have been suggested by many investigators as an opportunity to improve our ability to diagnose and treat stroke in a timely and safe manner [59].

Recent studies have indicated that the pathophysiological kinetics of serum GFAP, an intermediate filament protein expressed in astroglial cells, may render GFAP a promising contender in the search for acute biomarkers [47]. Trauma or disease-induced cellular necrosis in the brain and spinal cord are known to augment GFAP levels released into the plasma, and numerous findings have suggested that the more immediate structural damage to the artery and blood-brain barrier caused by hemorrhage in comparison with ischemic stroke renders the subsequent surge in GFAP levels a reliable indicator of hemorrhage specifically [60–63]. Within the first 6 h of stroke onset, significantly higher levels of serum GFAP have been found in patients suffering from hemorrhage than in those with ischemic stroke [62, 63]. Indeed, both GFAP and other biomarkers generally indicative of stress and morphological trauma, such as S100B, do not seem to peak until 2–4 days following ischemic stroke onset [63, 64]. In cases of hemorrhage, these levels decline roughly 6–12 h after symptom onset, within a time window before which biomarker surges are observed in ischemic stroke [63]. It should be noted, however, that S100B may not be as reliable and sensitive an indicator of hemorrhage as GFAP, as S100B levels are not necessarily as elevated within the first few hours of SAH as they are in intracerebral hemorrhage. Thus, diagnostic strategies employing GFAP would be expected to overlook fewer cases of hemorrhage. Moreover, serum GFAP levels have also accorded well with observational features, with this protein concentration directly proportional to acute stroke severity (as measured by NIHSS) and Intracranial Hemorrhage (ICH) volume and inversely proportional to functionality as long as 3 months after stroke onset. Cutoff points for serum GFAP level significance, however, have ranged from 0.29 to 2.9 μg/L [62, 63].

3. Biomarkers of neuronal injury

3.1. Neuron specific enolase (NSE)

Neuron specific enolase (NSE), an isozyme of the glycolytic enzyme enolase, is found in central and peripheral neuronal cell bodies. It increases in serum following cell injury [65] and has a biological half-life of 48 h. Notably, it is also present in erythrocytes and endocrine cells [66]. NSE is passively released into the extracellular space only under pathological conditions during cell destruction. Several studies have been published examining serum NSE following mild TBI [65, 67–70]. Many of these reports contained inadequate control groups and noted that serum NSE had limited utility as a marker of neuronal damage after trauma. Early levels of NSE concentrations have been correlated with outcome in children, particularly those under 4 years of age [71–74]. In the setting of diffuse axonal injury (DAI) in severe TBI, levels of NSE at 72 h of injury have shown an association with unfavorable outcome [75]. One of the limitations of NSE is the occurrence of false positive results in the setting of hemolysis [76, 77].

Data surrounding potential correlations between NSE concentration and ischemia are somewhat mixed and thus require continued research. Missler et al. found that serum concentrations of NSE in patients suffering from acute ischemia did increase, peaking on day 1.9 after onset and were significantly correlated with infarction volume as measured by CT [78]. NSE levels, however, were not found to correlate with outcome as determined by the GCS during either discharge or 6 months post onset [78]. Martens [79] studied NSE levels in patients who had lapsed into unconsciousness following acute global ischemia and found significant differences in serum and CSF NSE concentrations between those who regained consciousness and those who died or slipped into a vegetative state. Infants suffering from hypoxic ischemic encephalopathy (HIE) were marked by significantly increased concentrations of serum NSE 4–48 h and 5 days after birth, in comparison to healthy controls, and moreover expressed higher levels of NSE when suffering from the more severe stage III HIE rather than stages I or II, with NSE levels predicting poor outcome [80]. Jung et al., however, reported that while CSF NSE levels rose in response to SAH, they failed to correlate with the resulting cerebral vasospasm as glycine, glutamate, histidine, and glutamine did. Additionally, serum NSE levels failed to correlate with vasospasm development and ischemia in general [81]. In cases of hemorrhage, results about serum NSE were similarly mixed. Moritz et al. found that among patients who had suffered spontaneous SAH, both mean and peak concentrations of CSF but not serum NSE sampled within 8 days of onset predicted high or low performance on the GCS and predicted cerebral infarction and intracranial hypertension, but not vasospasm [82]. While Kuroiwa et al. did not observe a correlation between SAH and intracerebral hemorrhage patients' serum NSE concentrations and initial state of consciousness and neurological profile at admission, serum NSE levels tended to be higher in those with higher Fisher CT scores of 3 or 4 [83]. Moreover, those who were found to have vasospasm via cerebral angiography tended to experience peak NSE levels between days 5 and 15 since onset. Moreover, a correlation was observed between serum NSE level and hematoma size in those whose hematoma was 5 cm or greater [83]. Similarly, Oertel et al. found that SAH patients had higher levels of serum NSE within 3 days of onset if they had received Fisher CT scores of 4. However, unlike S100B, NSE was not found to reliably predict or be correlated with anything else, including vasospasm or GCS-determined outcome [84]. In terms of distinguishing between SAH and acute onset migraine, serum NSE levels were found to be significantly reduced in those with acute benign migraine in comparison to healthy controls, though they did not necessarily serve to indicate neurological injury [85].

3.2. Ubiquitin C-terminal hydrolase (UCH-L1)

A promising candidate biomarker for TBI currently under investigation is ubiquitin C-terminal hydrolase-L1 (UCH-L1). This protein is involved in the addition and removal of ubiquitin from proteins that are destined for metabolism [86] and therefore, has an important role in the removal of excessive, oxidized, or misfolded proteins in neurons [87]. UCH-L1 was previously used as a histological marker for neurons [88]. Clinical studies in humans with severe TBI have confirmed that the UCH-L1 protein is significantly elevated in human CSF and is detectable very early after injury [89, 90]. It remains significantly elevated for at least 1 week post injury [90] and there is very good correlation between CSF and serum levels [91]. Serum UCH-L1 is also elevated in children with moderate and severe TBI [92]. Most recently, UCH-L1 was detected in the serum of mild TBI patients within an hour of injury [47, 93]. Serum levels of UCH-L1 discriminated concussion patients from uninjured and non-head-injured trauma control patients who had orthopedic injuries or motor vehicle trauma without head injury [47, 93]. A handful of studies have shown serum UCH-L1 levels to be significantly higher in those with intracranial lesions on CT than those without lesions [45, 47, 93, 94] and to be much higher in those eventually requiring a neurosurgical intervention [47, 93]. The temporal profile of UCH-L1 was evaluated in a large cohort of 584 trauma patients seen at the emergency department. UCH-L1 rose rapidly and peaked at 8 h after injury and declined rapidly over 48 h [47].

Despite UCH-L1's capacity to identify concussive TBI, it is perhaps best employed prognostically, like S100B, in the assessment of stroke. Because increased serum and CSF concentrations of UCH-L1 are symptomatic of blood-brain barrier disruption, the deubiquinating enzyme is particularly useful in assessing both brain damage severity (i.e., infarction volume and extent of vasospasm) and the resulting outcome in patients who have suffered hemorrhage or ischemia. Indeed, studies investigating the role of UCH-L1 in stroke have noted its potential to measure neurodegenerative injury. Individuals who suffered acute ischemic episodes within 12–24 h following an aortic aneurysm repair were found to have elevated CSF concentrations of UCH-L1 [95]. Despite the confounders of surgical distress and cardiopulmonary or circulatory complication, the study concluded that UCH-L1 levels were reliably associated with neurological damage. The 12–24 h timescale restricts the use of UCH-L1 to monitoring, even though ischemic apoptosis has been noted to peak at 24–48 h post onset [47–95]. UCH-L1 holds therapeutic promise for ischemia patients to the extent that it and similar deubiquinating enzymes have been found to reduce infarction in cases of rapid ischemic tolerance following brief ischemia [96]. Interestingly, polyubiquinated protein buildups in hippocampal synapses have been reported in response to global ischemia [97], raising the question of how well such results might coordinate with MRI imaging data. The potential role of UCH-L1 in cases of hemorrhage is perhaps clearer. Lewis et al. found that individuals suffering from aneurysmal (SAH) had consistently higher concentrations of UCH-L1 in the CSF 2 weeks after post-aneurysmal rupture, which moreover were significantly associated with poor recovery [98]. Furthermore, patients in whom CSF S100B levels reduced experienced improved recovery when UCH-L1 concentrations dropped as well. Siman et al. similarly found that CSF concentrations of UCH-L1, among an array of seven other biomarkers including NSE and S100B, taken over a 10-day period since aneurysmal rupture, rose significantly and predicted severity of infarction, vasospasm, and outcome [95]. However, they found mixed results for whether UCH-L1 levels peaked on the first day, the seventh day, or remained relatively consistent throughout the measured time course.

4. Biomarkers of axonal injury

4.1. Alpha-II spectrin breakdown products

Alpha-II-spectrin is a 280-kDa protein that is an important structural component of the cortical membrane cytoskeleton, particularly abundant in axons and presynaptic terminals [99, 100]. It serves as is a key substrate for both calpain-2 and caspase-3 cysteine proteases [101, 102]. These proteases (caspase-3 and calpain-2) cleave cytoskeletal αII-spectrin [103, 104] into spectrin breakdown products (SBDPs). These SBDPs have been reported in CSF from adults with severe TBI and they have shown a significant relationship with severity of injury and clinical outcome [105–112]. The time course of calpain-mediated SBDP150 and SBDP145 (markers of necrosis) differs from that of caspase-3-mediated SBDP120 (marker of apoptosis) and have been shown to correlate with severity of injury, CT scan findings, and outcome at 6 months post injury [111, 112]. These findings were similar in children with moderate to severe TBI [92]. More recently, serum levels of SBDP150 measured in mild TBI patients have shown a significant association with acute measures of injury severity, such as GCS score, intracranial injuries on CT, and neurosurgical intervention [113]. In this study, serum SBDP150 levels were much higher in patients with concussion than other trauma patients who did not have a head injury [113].

In patients suffering from aneurysmal subarachnoid hemorrhage, CSF concentrations of calpain-mediated and caspase-mediated SBDPs have been found to be significantly elevated within 72 h post onset and up to 12 h pre-cerebral arterial vasospasm due to the role of necrotic proteolysis in hemorrhage and vasospasm-induced neurodegeneration [114, 115]. Research on the potential role of SBDPs in human ischemia has been comparatively more sparse, though rat studies have indicated an association between caspase-mediated spectrin breakdown products and ischemia-induced apoptosis [116, 117], and the overstimulation of mammalian calpain 1 and calpain 2 has been understood to be involved with the pathophysiology of acute stroke [118]. Moreover, alpha-spectrin-related insights into treatment potential for both cerebral ischemia and TBI have surfaced in the form of caspase cascade inhibitors, which have been able to arrest processes of apoptosis in the aftermath of the aforementioned acute neurological disorders [119, 120]. Biomarker panel including assays of caspase-3 and D-dimer has potential in delineating stroke from ischemic stroke mimics, such as acute migraine [121].

4.2. Tau protein

Tau is an intracellular, microtubule-associated protein that is highly enriched in axons and is involved with assembling axonal microtubule bundles and participating in anterograde axoplasmic transport [122]. Tau lesions are apparently related to axonal disruption such as in trauma or hypoxia [123, 124]. After release, it is proteolytically cleaved at the N- and C-terminals. The C-tau has been investigated as a potential biomarker of CNS injury.

Initial elevated CSF C-tau levels in severe TBI patients have been shown to predict elevations in intracranial pressure and to be associated with poor clinical outcome [125]. In a study by Shaw et al., an elevated level of C-tau was associated with a poor outcome at hospital discharge and with an increased chance of an intracranial injury on head CT [126]. However, these findings were not reproducible when C-tau was measured in peripheral blood in mild TBI [127]. Two additional studies showed that C-tau was a poor predictor of CT lesions and a poor predictor of post-concussive syndrome [15, 128]. Total tau (T-tau) has also been found to be correlated with severity of injury in severe TBI [129–132]. Ost et al. found that tau measured in CSF on days 2 to 3 discriminated between TBI and controls with (normal pressure hydrocephalus) and also between good and bad outcome at 1 year per dichotomized Glasgow Outcome Scale (GOS) score [131]. Unfortunately, T-tau was not detected in serum throughout the study. Phosphorylated -tau (P-Tau) is also being examined following head trauma [133].

The hyperphosphorylation of tau in the development of apoptosis-related neurofibrillary tangles has been explored in relation to neurodegeneration induced by transient cerebral ischemia [134]. Dewar et al. suggested the role of cytoskeletal breakdown in both cerebral focal ischemia and Alzheimer's-induced impairment, having found that permanent focal cerebral ischemia resulted in modification of the protein tau [135]. Results have been more prolific for hemorrhage, perhaps due to the more immediate severity and thus morphological damage it tends to entail. In accordance with the aforementioned time scale for TBI, Hu et al. observed that serum tau levels in patients with intracerebral hemorrhage were significantly predictive of 3-month mortality, with these prognoses achieving greater predictive accuracy than the NIHSS [136]. Augmented CSF levels of tau were reported in patients following severe episodes of aneurysmal subarachnoid hemorrhage in comparison with more moderate episodes, also correlating with the motor score on the GCS and proving more elevated in those patients with fatal outcomes [137].

4.3. Neurofilaments

Neurofilaments are heteropolymeric components of the neuron cytoskeleton that consist of a 68-kDa light neurofilament subunit (NF-L) backbone with either 160 kDa medium (NF-M) or 200 kDa heavy subunit (NF-H) side arms [138]. They provide structural support for the axon. It is postulated that after a TBI, calcineurin (a calcium-dependent phosphatase) dephosphorylates neurofilament side arms, and contributes to axonal injury [139]. Phosphorylated NF-H in CSF has been found to be elevated in adult patients with severe TBI compared to controls [89]. Hyperphosphorylated NF-H has also been correlated with severity of brain injury in children [140]. In this study, NF-H levels taken on the second to fourth day remained significantly higher in patients with poor outcome in comparison to patients with good outcome and in those children with DAI on initial CT scan [140]. Vajtr et al. also found elevated serum NF-H in patients with DAI over 10 days after admission with highest levels from day 4 to 10 [141].

Serum concentrations of phosphorylated NFL-H (pNFL-H) sampled from patients with acute ischemia have been shown to correlate with CT scan assessment of ischemia upon admission and at 7 days post onset as determined by the Alberta Stroke Program Early CT Scale, NIHSS, and GCS [142]. Sellner et al. also found significantly higher serum pNFL-H concentrations in ischemic patients 24 h after onset [143]. However, exploration of the timely diagnostic value of pNFL-H for ischemia has again been mixed. While Singh et al. observed elevation of serum pNFL-H in ischemic patients, levels did not reach significance or predict patient outcome or infarct volume until 3 weeks post onset [144]. In cases of hemorrhagic stroke, neurofilaments show promise as prognostic markers, with elevated CSF levels assayed within 10–14 days of aneurysmal SAH onset and correlating with GCS performance as 1 year post onset [145]. Assays of pNFL-H were also found to correlate with early neurological deterioration and survival rates 6 months post onset with accuracy comparable to that of the NIHSS [146].

5. Conclusion

There is a great need to validate brain injury biofluid biomarkers in the acute care setting such as in the emergency department. Biomarkers measured through a simple blood test have the potential to provide invaluable information about the management of acute brain injury for

http://dx.doi.org/10.5772/64222

conditions such as TBI and stroke. Biomarkers could potentially facilitate diagnosis and risk stratification of these patients. Biomarkers could provide timely information about the pathophysiology of injury to allow for monitoring and assessment of progression and recovery. Biomarkers could provide major opportunities for drug target identification and guide the conduct of clinical research as surrogate outcome measures. Although research in the field of brain injury biomarkers has increased significantly over the last decade, clinical studies have not been adequately powered with enough patients to validate them. Large clinical studies are underway that will change this and will bring a blood test closer to the bedside.

Author details

Linda Papa* and Kimberly Rosenthal

*Address all correspondence to: lpstat@aol.com

Department of Emergency Medicine, Orlando Regional Medical Center, Orlando, FL, USA

References

[1] Papa L, Edwards D, Ramia M. Exploring serum biomarkers for mild traumatic brain injury. *In: Brain Injury Principles: Molecular, Neuropsychological, and Rehabilitation Aspects in Brain Injury Models.* CRC Press/Taylor & Francis (Boca Raton, FL). E-Pub August 14, 2015

[2] Papa L, Ramia MM, Edwards D, Johnson BD, Slobounov SM. Systematic review of clinical studies examining biomarkers of brain injury in athletes after sports-related concussion. J Neurotrauma 2015;32:661–73.

[3] Papa L, Ramia MM, Kelly JM, Burks SS, Pawlowicz A, Berger RP. Systematic review of clinical research on biomarkers for pediatric traumatic brain injury. J Neurotrauma 2013;30:324–38.

[4] Papa L, Robinson G, Oli M, et al. Use of biomarkers for diagnosis and management of traumatic brain injury patients. Expert Opin Med Diagn 2008;2:937–45.

[5] Xiong H, Liang WL, Wu XR. Pathophysiological alterations in cultured astrocytes exposed to hypoxia/reoxygenation. Sheng Li Ke Xue Jin Zhan 2000;31:217–21.

[6] Zimmer DB, Cornwall EH, Landar A, Song W. The S100 protein family: history, function, and expression. Brain Res Bull 1995;37:417–29.

[7] Olsson B, Zetterberg H, Hampel H, Blennow K. Biomarker-based dissection of neurodegenerative diseases. Prog Neurobiol 2011;95:520–34.

[8] Schulte S, Podlog LW, Hamson-Utley JJ, Strathmann FG, Struder HK. A systematic review of the biomarker S100B: implications for sport-related concussion management. J Athl Train 2014;49:830–50.

[9] Ingebrigtsen T, Romner B. Management of minor head injuries in hospitals in Norway. Acta Neurol Scand 1997;95:51–5.

[10] Waterloo K, Ingebrigtsen T, Romner B. Neuropsychological function in patients with increased serum levels of protein S-100 after minor head injury. Acta Neurochir (Wien) 1997;139:26–31; discussion -2.

[11] Ingebrigtsen T, Romner B. Serial S-100 protein serum measurements related to early magnetic resonance imaging after minor head injury. Case report. J Neurosurg 1996;85:945–8.

[12] Ingebrigtsen T, Waterloo K, Jacobsen EA, Langbakk B, Romner B. Traumatic brain damage in minor head injury: relation of serum S-100 protein measurements to magnetic resonance imaging and neurobehavioral outcome. Neurosurgery 1999;45:468–75; discussion 75–6.

[13] Heidari K, Asadollahi S, Jamshidian M, Abrishamchi SN, Nouroozi M. Prediction of neuropsychological outcome after mild traumatic brain injury using clinical parameters, serum S100B protein and findings on computed tomography. Brain Inj 2015;29:33–40.

[14] Metting Z, Wilczak N, Rodiger LA, Schaaf JM, van der Naalt J. GFAP and S100B in the acute phase of mild traumatic brain injury. Neurology 2012;78:1428–33.

[15] Bazarian JJ, Zemlan FP, Mookerjee S, Stigbrand T. Serum S-100B and cleaved-tau are poor predictors of long-term outcome after mild traumatic brain injury. Brain Inj 2006;20:759–65.

[16] Lima DP, Simao Filho C, Abib Sde C, de Figueiredo LF. Quality of life and neuropsychological changes in mild head trauma. Late analysis and correlation with S100B protein and cranial CT scan performed at hospital admission. Injury 2008;39:604–11.

[17] Dorminy M, Hoogeveen A, Tierney RT, Higgins M, McDevitt JK, Kretzschmar J. Effect of soccer heading ball speed on S100B, sideline concussion assessments and head impact kinematics. Brain Inj 2015:1–7.

[18] Heidari K, Vafaee A, Rastekenari AM, et al. S100B protein as a screening tool for computed tomography findings after mild traumatic brain injury: systematic review and meta-analysis. Brain Inj 2015:1–12.

[19] Pelinka LE, Kroepfl A, Schmidhammer R, et al. Glial fibrillary acidic protein in serum after traumatic brain injury and multiple trauma. J Trauma 2004;57:1006–12.

[20] Papa L, Mittal MK, Ramirez J, et al. In children and youth with mild and moderate traumatic brain injury, glial fibrillary acidic protein out-performs S100beta in detecting

traumatic intracranial lesions on computed tomography. J Neurotrauma 2016;33:58–64.

[21] Papa L, Silvestri S, Brophy GM, et al. GFAP out-performs S100beta in detecting traumatic intracranial lesions on computed tomography in trauma patients with mild traumatic brain injury and those with extracranial lesions. J Neurotrauma 2014;31:1815–22.

[22] Fassbender K, Schmidt R, Schreiner A, et al. Leakage of brain-originated proteins in peripheral blood: temporal profile and diagnostic value in early ischemic stroke. J Neurol Sci 1997;148:101–5.

[23] Nafria C, Fernandez-Cadenas I, Mendioroz M, et al. Update on the serum biomarkers and genetic factors associated with safety and efficacy of rt-PA treatment in acute stroke patients. Stroke Res Treat 2011;2011:182783.

[24] Kennedy MS, Ferri RS, Sofer D. tPA after stroke: the sooner the better: clinical benefit is gone by six hours. Am J Nurs 2004;104:18.

[25] Barbieri A, Giuliani E, Carone C, et al. Clinical severity of ischemic stroke and neural damage biomarkers in the acute setting: the STROke MArkers (STROMA) study. Minerva Anestesiol 2013;79:750–7.

[26] Amar AP. Brain and vascular imaging of acute stroke. World Neurosurg 2012;76:S3–8.

[27] Rodriguez-Yanez M, Sobrino T, Arias S, et al. Early biomarkers of clinical-diffusion mismatch in acute ischemic stroke. Stroke 2011;42:2813–8.

[28] Schellinger PD, Latour LL, Wu CS, Chalela JA, Warach S. The association between neurological deficit in acute ischemic stroke and mean transit time: comparison of four different perfusion MRI algorithms. Neuroradiology 2006;48:69–77.

[29] Kang DW, Chalela JA, Dunn W, Warach S. MRI screening before standard tissue plasminogen activator therapy is feasible and safe. Stroke 2005;36:1939–43.

[30] Kidwell CS, Chalela JA, Saver JL, et al. Comparison of MRI and CT for detection of acute intracerebral hemorrhage. JAMA 2004;292:1823–30.

[31] Teepker M, Munk K, Mylius V, et al. Serum concentrations of s100b and NSE in migraine. Headache 2009;49:245–52.

[32] Papandreou O, Soldatou A, Tsitsika A, et al. Serum S100beta protein in children with acute recurrent headache: a potentially useful marker for migraine. Headache 2005;45:1313–6.

[33] Eng LF, Vanderhaeghen JJ, Bignami A, Gerstl B. An acidic protein isolated from fibrous astrocytes. Brain Res 1971;28:351–4.

[34] Duchen LW. General pathology of neurons and neuroglia. In: Adams JA, Corsellis JAN, Duchen LW, eds. Greenfield's Neuropathology. London: Edward Arnold; 1984:1–52.

[35] Baydas G, Nedzvetskii VS, Tuzcu M, Yasar A, Kirichenko SV. Increase of glial fibrillary acidic protein and S-100B in hippocampus and cortex of diabetic rats: effects of vitamin E. Eur J Pharmacol 2003;462:67–71.

[36] Mouser PE, Head E, Ha KH, Rohn TT. Caspase-mediated cleavage of glial fibrillary acidic protein within degenerating astrocytes of the Alzheimer's disease brain. Am J Pathol 2006;168:936–46.

[37] Herrmann M, Vos P, Wunderlich MT, de Bruijn CH, Lamers KJ. Release of glial tissue-specific proteins after acute stroke: a comparative analysis of serum concentrations of protein S-100B and glial fibrillary acidic protein. Stroke 2000;31:2670–7.

[38] Missler U, Wiesmann M, Wittmann G, Magerkurth O, Hagenstrom H. Measurement of glial fibrillary acidic protein in human blood: analytical method and preliminary clinical results. Clin Chem 1999;45:138–41.

[39] Pelinka LE, Kroepfl A, Leixnering M, Buchinger W, Raabe A, Redl H. GFAP versus S100B in serum after traumatic brain injury: relationship to brain damage and outcome. J Neurotrauma 2004;21:1553–61.

[40] van Geel WJ, de Reus HP, Nijzing H, Verbeek MM, Vos PE, Lamers KJ. Measurement of glial fibrillary acidic protein in blood: an analytical method. Clin Chim Acta 2002;326:151–4.

[41] Nylen K, Ost M, Csajbok LZ, et al. Increased serum-GFAP in patients with severe traumatic brain injury is related to outcome. J Neurol Sci 2006;240:85–91.

[42] Mondello S, Papa L, Buki A, et al. Neuronal and glial markers are differently associated with computed tomography findings and outcome in patients with severe traumatic brain injury: a case control study. Crit Care 2011;15:R156.

[43] Vos PE, Jacobs B, Andriessen TM, et al. GFAP and S100B are biomarkers of traumatic brain injury: an observational cohort study. Neurology 2010;75:1786–93.

[44] Papa L, Lewis LM, Falk JL, et al. Elevated levels of serum glial fibrillary acidic protein breakdown products in mild and moderate traumatic brain injury are associated with intracranial lesions and neurosurgical intervention. Ann Emerg Med 2012;59:471–83.

[45] Diaz-Arrastia R, Wang KK, Papa L, et al. Acute biomarkers of traumatic brain injury: relationship between plasma levels of ubiquitin C-terminal hydrolase-L1 and glial fibrillary acidic protein. J Neurotrauma 2014;31:19–25.

[46] Papa L, Zonfrillo MR, Ramirez J, et al. Performance of glial fibrillary acidic protein in detecting traumatic intracranial lesions on computed tomography in children and youth with mild head trauma. Acad Emerg Med 2015;22:1274–82.

[47] Papa L, Brophy GM, Welch RD, et al. Time course and diagnostic accuracy of glial and neuronal blood biomarkers GFAP and UCH-L1 in a large cohort of trauma patients with and without mild traumatic brain injury. JAMA Neurol 2016;73:551-60.

[48] Marks MP, Olivot JM, Kemp S, et al. Patients with acute stroke treated with intravenous tPA 3-6 hours after stroke onset: correlations between MR angiography findings and perfusion- and diffusion-weighted imaging in the DEFUSE study. Radiology 2008;249:614–23.

[49] Thomalla G, Schwark C, Sobesky J, et al. Outcome and symptomatic bleeding complications of intravenous thrombolysis within 6 hours in MRI-selected stroke patients: comparison of a German multicenter study with the pooled data of ATLANTIS, ECASS, and NINDS tPA trials. Stroke 2006;37:852–8.

[50] Chen CH, Tang SC, Tsai LK, et al. Stroke code improves intravenous thrombolysis administration in acute ischemic stroke. PLoS One 2014;9:e104862.

[51] Uchino K, Alexandrov AV, Garami Z, El-Mitwalli A, Morgenstern LB, Grotta JC. Safety and feasibility of a lower dose intravenous TPA therapy for ischemic stroke beyond the first three hours. Cerebrovasc Dis 2005;19:260–6.

[52] Campbell BC, Mitchell PJ, Yan B, et al. A multicenter, randomized, controlled study to investigate EXtending the time for Thrombolysis in Emergency Neurological Deficits with Intra-Arterial therapy (EXTEND-IA). Int J Stroke 2014;9:126–32.

[53] Goyal M, Demchuk AM, Menon BK, et al. Randomized assessment of rapid endovascular treatment of ischemic stroke. N Engl J Med 2015;372:1019–30.

[54] Berkhemer OA, Fransen PS, Beumer D, et al. A randomized trial of intraarterial treatment for acute ischemic stroke. N Engl J Med 2015;372:11–20.

[55] Yilmaz A, Akpinar E, Topcuoglu MA, Arsava EM. Clinical and imaging features associated with intracranial internal carotid artery calcifications in patients with ischemic stroke. Neuroradiology 2015;57:501–6.

[56] Grysiewicz RA, Thomas K, Pandey DK. Epidemiology of ischemic and hemorrhagic stroke: incidence, prevalence, mortality, and risk factors. Neurol Clin 2008;26:871–95, vii.

[57] Kang DW, Latour LL, Chalela JA, Dambrosia JA, Warach S. Early and late recurrence of ischemic lesion on MRI: evidence for a prolonged stroke-prone state? Neurology 2004;63:2261–5.

[58] Chalela JA, Kang DW, Warach S. Multiple cerebral microbleeds: MRI marker of a diffuse hemorrhage-prone state. J Neuroimaging 2004;14:54–7.

[59] Oliver WJ, Shope TC, Kuhns LR. Fatal lumbar puncture: fact versus fiction – an approach to a clinical dilemma. Pediatrics 2003;112:e174–6.

[60] Mohr JP, Kejda-Scharler J. A strong start: plasma glial fibrillary acidic protein and stroke differential diagnosis. Clin Chem 2011;58:319–20.

[61] Jensen MB, Chacon MR, Sattin JA, Aleu A, Lyden PD. The promise and potential pitfalls of serum biomarkers for ischemic stroke and transient ischemic attack. Neurologist 2008;14:243–6.

[62] Foerch C, Curdt I, Yan B, et al. Serum glial fibrillary acidic protein as a biomarker for intracerebral haemorrhage in patients with acute stroke. J Neurol Neurosurg Psychiatry 2006;77:181–4.

[63] Foerch C, Niessner M, Back T, et al. Diagnostic accuracy of plasma glial fibrillary acidic protein for differentiating intracerebral hemorrhage and cerebral ischemia in patients with symptoms of acute stroke. Clin Chem 2012;58:237–45.

[64] Wunderlich MT, Wallesch CW, Goertler M. Release of glial fibrillary acidic protein is related to the neurovascular status in acute ischemic stroke. Eur J Neurol 2006;13:1118–23.

[65] Skogseid IM, Nordby HK, Urdal P, Paus E, Lilleaas F. Increased serum creatine kinase BB and neuron specific enolase following head injury indicates brain damage. Acta Neurochir (Wien) 1992;115:106–11.

[66] Schmechel D, Marangos PJ, Brightman M. Neurone-specific enolase is a molecular marker for peripheral and central neuroendocrine cells. Nature 1978;276:834–6.

[67] Ergun R, Bostanci U, Akdemir G, et al. Prognostic value of serum neuron-specific enolase levels after head injury. Neurol Res 1998;20:418–20.

[68] Yamazaki Y, Yada K, Morii S, Kitahara T, Ohwada T. Diagnostic significance of serum neuron-specific enolase and myelin basic protein assay in patients with acute head injury. Surg Neurol 1995;43:267–70; discussion 70–1.

[69] Ross SA, Cunningham RT, Johnston CF, Rowlands BJ. Neuron-specific enolase as an aid to outcome prediction in head injury. Br J Neurosurg 1996;10:471–6.

[70] Fridriksson T, Kini N, Walsh-Kelly C, Hennes H. Serum neuron-specific enolase as a predictor of intracranial lesions in children with head trauma: a pilot study. Acad Emerg Med 2000;7:816–20.

[71] Berger RP, Adelson PD, Pierce MC, Dulani T, Cassidy LD, Kochanek PM. Serum neuron-specific enolase, S100B, and myelin basic protein concentrations after inflicted and noninflicted traumatic brain injury in children. J Neurosurg 2005;103:61–8.

[72] Berger RP, Beers SR, Richichi R, Wiesman D, Adelson PD. Serum biomarker concentrations and outcome after pediatric traumatic brain injury. J Neurotrauma 2007;24:1793–801.

[73] Varma S, Janesko KL, Wisniewski SR, et al. F2-isoprostane and neuron-specific enolase in cerebrospinal fluid after severe traumatic brain injury in infants and children. J Neurotrauma 2003;20:781–6.

[74] Bandyopadhyay S, Hennes H, Gorelick MH, Wells RG, Walsh-Kelly CM. Serum neuron-specific enolase as a predictor of short-term outcome in children with closed traumatic brain injury. Acad Emerg Med 2005;12:732–8.

[75] Chabok SY, Moghadam AD, Saneei Z, Amlashi FG, Leili EK, Amiri ZM. Neuron-specific enolase and S100BB as outcome predictors in severe diffuse axonal injury. J Trauma Acute Care Surg 2012;72:1654–7.

[76] Johnsson P, Blomquist S, Luhrs C, et al. Neuron-specific enolase increases in plasma during and immediately after extracorporeal circulation. Ann Thorac Surg 2000;69:750–4.

[77] Ramont L, Thoannes H, Volondat A, Chastang F, Millet MC, Maquart FX. Effects of hemolysis and storage condition on neuron-specific enolase (NSE) in cerebrospinal fluid and serum: implications in clinical practice. Clin Chem Lab Med 2005;43:1215–7.

[78] Missler U, Wiesmann M, Friedrich C, Kaps M. S-100 protein and neuron-specific enolase concentrations in blood as indicators of infarction volume and prognosis in acute ischemic stroke. Stroke 1997;28:1956–60.

[79] Martens P. Serum neuron-specific enolase as a prognostic marker for irreversible brain damage in comatose cardiac arrest survivors. Acad Emerg Med 1996;3:126–31.

[80] Celtik C, Acunas B, Oner N, Pala O. Neuron-specific enolase as a marker of the severity and outcome of hypoxic ischemic encephalopathy. Brain Dev 2004;26:398–402.

[81] Jung CS, Lange B, Zimmermann M, Seifert V. CSF and serum biomarkers focusing on cerebral vasospasm and ischemia after subarachnoid hemorrhage. Stroke Res Treat 2013;2013:560305.

[82] Moritz S, Warnat J, Bele S, Graf BM, Woertgen C. The prognostic value of NSE and S100B from serum and cerebrospinal fluid in patients with spontaneous subarachnoid hemorrhage. J Neurosurg Anesthesiol 2009;22:21–31.

[83] Kuroiwa T, Tanabe H, Arai M, Ohta T. [Measurement of serum neuron-specific enolase levels after subarachnoid hemorrhage and intracerebral hemorrhage]. No Shinkei Geka 1994;22:531–5.

[84] Oertel M, Schumacher U, McArthur DL, Kastner S, Boker DK. S-100B and NSE: markers of initial impact of subarachnoid haemorrhage and their relation to vasospasm and outcome. J Clin Neurosci 2006;13:834–40.

[85] Casmiro M, Scarpa E, Cortelli P, Vignatelli L. Cerebrospinal fluid and serum neuron-specific enolase in acute benign headache. Cephalalgia 2008;28:506–9.

[86] Tongaonkar P, Chen L, Lambertson D, Ko B, Madura K. Evidence for an interaction between ubiquitin-conjugating enzymes and the 26S proteasome. Mol Cell Biol 2000;20:4691–8.

[87] Gong B, Leznik E. The role of ubiquitin C-terminal hydrolase L1 in neurodegenerative disorders. Drug News Perspect 2007;20:365–70.

[88] Jackson P, Thompson RJ. The demonstration of new human brain-specific proteins by high-resolution two-dimensional polyacrylamide gel electrophoresis. J Neurol Sci 1981;49:429–38.

[89] Siman R, Toraskar N, Dang A, et al. A panel of neuron-enriched proteins as markers for traumatic brain injury in humans. J Neurotrauma 2009;26:1867–77.

[90] Papa L, Akinyi L, Liu MC, et al. Ubiquitin C-terminal hydrolase is a novel biomarker in humans for severe traumatic brain injury. Crit Care Med 2010;38:138–44.

[91] Brophy G, Mondello S, Papa L, et al. Biokinetic analysis of ubiquitin C-terminal hydrolase-L1 (Uch-L1) in severe traumatic brain injury patient biofluids. J Neurotrauma.

[92] Berger RP, Beers SR, Papa L, Bell M. Common data elements for pediatric traumatic brain injury: recommendations from the biospecimens and biomarkers workgroup. J Neurotrauma 2012;29:672–7.

[93] Papa L, Lewis LM, Silvestri S, et al. Serum levels of ubiquitin C-terminal hydrolase distinguish mild traumatic brain injury from trauma controls and are elevated in mild and moderate traumatic brain injury patients with intracranial lesions and neurosurgical intervention. J Trauma Acute Care Surg 2012;72:1335–44.

[94] Welch RD, Ayaz SI, Lewis LM, et al. Ability of serum glial fibrillary acidic protein, ubiquitin C-terminal hydrolase-L1, and S100B to differentiate normal and abnormal head computed tomography findings in patients with suspected mild or moderate traumatic brain injury. J Neurotrauma 2015;33:203-14.

[95] Siman R, Giovannone N, Toraskar N, et al. Evidence that a panel of neurodegeneration biomarkers predicts vasospasm, infarction, and outcome in aneurysmal subarachnoid hemorrhage. PLoS One 2011;6:e28938.

[96] Meller R. The role of the ubiquitin proteasome system in ischemia and ischemic tolerance. Neuroscientist 2009;15:243–60.

[97] Liu MC, Akinyi L, Scharf D, et al. Ubiquitin C-terminal hydrolase-L1 as a biomarker for ischemic and traumatic brain injury in rats. Eur J Neurosci 2010;31:722–32.

[98] Lewis SB, Wolper R, Chi YY, et al. Identification and preliminary characterization of ubiquitin C terminal hydrolase 1 (UCHL1) as a biomarker of neuronal loss in aneurysmal subarachnoid hemorrhage. J Neurosci Res 2010;88:1475–84.

[99] Goodman SR, Zimmer WE, Clark MB, Zagon IS, Barker JE, Bloom ML. Brain spectrin: of mice and men. Brain Res Bull 1995;36:593–606.

[100] Riederer BM, Zagon IS, Goodman SR. Brain spectrin(240/235) and brain spectrin(240/235E): two distinct spectrin subtypes with different locations within mammalian neural cells. J Cell Biol 1986;102:2088–97.

[101] Wang KK, Posmantur R, Nath R, et al. Simultaneous degradation of alphaII- and betaII-spectrin by caspase 3 (CPP32) in apoptotic cells. J Biol Chem 1998;273:22490–7.

[102] McGinn MJ, Kelley BJ, Akinyi L, et al. Biochemical, structural, and biomarker evidence for calpain-mediated cytoskeletal change after diffuse brain injury uncomplicated by contusion. J Neuropathol Exp Neurol 2009;68:241–9.

[103] Pike BR, Flint J, Dave JR, et al. Accumulation of calpain and caspase-3 proteolytic fragments of brain-derived alphaII-spectrin in cerebral spinal fluid after middle cerebral artery occlusion in rats. J Cereb Blood Flow Metab 2004;24:98–106.

[104] Ringger NC, O'Steen BE, Brabham JG, et al. A novel marker for traumatic brain injury: CSF alphaII-spectrin breakdown product levels. J Neurotrauma 2004;21:1443–56.

[105] Cardali S, Maugeri R. Detection of alphaII-spectrin and breakdown products in humans after severe traumatic brain injury. J Neurosurg Sci 2006;50:25–31.

[106] Pineda JA, Lewis SB, Valadka AB, et al. Clinical significance of alphaII-spectrin breakdown products in cerebrospinal fluid after severe traumatic brain injury. J Neurotrauma 2007;24:354–66.

[107] Papa L, D'Avella D, Aguennouz M, et al. Detection of alpha-II spectrin and breakdown products in humans after severe traumatic brain injury [abstract]. Acad Emerg Med 2004;11 (5): 515.

[108] Papa L, Lewis SB, Heaton S, et al. Predicting early outcome using alpha-II spectrin breakdown products in human CSF after severe traumatic brain injury [abstract]. Acad Emerg Med 2006;13 (5) Suppl 1:S39-S40.

[109] Papa L, Pineda J, Wang KKW, et al. Levels of alpha-II spectrin breakdown products in human CSF and outcome after severe traumatic brain injury [abstract]. Acad Emerg Med 2005;12 (5) Suppl 1: 139-140.

[110] Mondello S, Robicsek SA, Gabrielli A, et al. alphaII-spectrin breakdown products (SBDPs): diagnosis and outcome in severe traumatic brain injury patients. J Neurotrauma 2010;27:1203–13.

[111] Brophy GM, Pineda JA, Papa L, et al. alphaII-Spectrin breakdown product cerebrospinal fluid exposure metrics suggest differences in cellular injury mechanisms after severe traumatic brain injury. J Neurotrauma 2009;26:471–9.

[112] Papa L, Robertson CS, Wang KK, et al. Biomarkers improve clinical outcome predictors of mortality following non-penetrating severe traumatic brain injury. Neurocrit Care 2015;22:52–64.

[113] Papa L, Wang KW, G.B. B, et al. Serum Levels of Spectrin Breakdown Product 150 (SBDP150) distinguish Mild Traumatic Brain Injury from Trauma and Uninjured

Controls and Predict Intracranial Injuries on CT and Neurosurgical Intervention. J Neurotrauma 2012;29:A28.

[114] Lewis SB, Velat GJ, Miralia L, et al. Alpha-II spectrin breakdown products in aneurysmal subarachnoid hemorrhage: a novel biomarker of proteolytic injury. J Neurosurg 2007;107:792–6.

[115] Nath R, Huggins M, Glantz SB, et al. Development and characterization of antibodies specific to caspase-3-produced alpha II-spectrin 120 kDa breakdown product: marker for neuronal apoptosis. Neurochem Int 2000;37:351–61.

[116] Siman R, Zhang C, Roberts VL, Pitts-Kiefer A, Neumar RW. Novel surrogate markers for acute brain damage: cerebrospinal fluid levels correlate with severity of ischemic neurodegeneration in the rat. J Cereb Blood Flow Metab 2005;25:1433–44.

[117] Zhang C, Siman R, Xu YA, Mills AM, Frederick JR, Neumar RW. Comparison of calpain and caspase activities in the adult rat brain after transient forebrain ischemia. Neurobiol Dis 2002;10:289–05.

[118] Huang Y, Wang KK. The calpain family and human disease. Trends Mol Med 2001;7:355–62.

[119] Fasulo L, Ugolini G, Visintin M, et al. The neuronal microtubule-associated protein tau is a substrate for caspase-3 and an effector of apoptosis. J Neurochem 2000;75:624–33.

[120] Lin HJ, Shaffer KM, Chang YH, et al. Acute exposure of toluene transiently potentiates p42/44 mitogen-activated protein kinase (MAPK) activity in cultured rat cortical astrocytes. Neurosci Lett 2002;332:103–6.

[121] Montaner J, Mendioroz M, Ribo M, et al. A panel of biomarkers including caspase-3 and D-dimer may differentiate acute stroke from stroke-mimicking conditions in the emergency department. J Intern Med 2011;270:166–74.

[122] Teunissen CE, Dijkstra C, Polman C. Biological markers in CSF and blood for axonal degeneration in multiple sclerosis. Lancet Neurol 2005;4:32–41.

[123] Kosik KS, Finch EA. MAP2 and tau segregate into dendritic and axonal domains after the elaboration of morphologically distinct neurites: an immunocytochemical study of cultured rat cerebrum. J Neurosci 1987;7:3142–53.

[124] Higuchi M, Lee VM, Trojanowski JQ. Tau and axonopathy in neurodegenerative disorders. Neuromolecular Med 2002;2:131–50.

[125] Zemlan FP, Jauch EC, Mulchahey JJ, et al. C-tau biomarker of neuronal damage in severe brain injured patients: association with elevated intracranial pressure and clinical outcome. Brain Res 2002;947:131–9.

[126] Shaw GJ, Jauch EC, Zemlan FP. Serum cleaved tau protein levels and clinical outcome in adult patients with closed head injury. Ann Emerg Med 2002;39:254–7.

[127] Chatfield DA, Zemlan FP, Day DJ, Menon DK. Discordant temporal patterns of S100beta and cleaved tau protein elevation after head injury: a pilot study. Br J Neurosurg 2002;16:471–6.

[128] Ma M, Lindsell CJ, Rosenberry CM, Shaw GJ, Zemlan FP. Serum cleaved tau does not predict postconcussion syndrome after mild traumatic brain injury. Am J Emerg Med 2008;26:763–8.

[129] Franz G, Beer R, Kampfl A, et al. Amyloid beta 1-42 and tau in cerebrospinal fluid after severe traumatic brain injury. Neurology 2003;60:1457–61.

[130] Marklund N, Blennow K, Zetterberg H, Ronne-Engstrom E, Enblad P, Hillered L. Monitoring of brain interstitial total tau and beta amyloid proteins by microdialysis in patients with traumatic brain injury. J Neurosurg 2009;110:1227–37.

[131] Ost M, Nylen K, Csajbok L, et al. Initial CSF total tau correlates with 1-year outcome in patients with traumatic brain injury. Neurology 2006;67:1600–4.

[132] Sjogren M, Blomberg M, Jonsson M, et al. Neurofilament protein in cerebrospinal fluid: a marker of white matter changes. J Neurosci Res 2001;66:510–6.

[133] Puvenna V, Engeler M, Banjara M, et al. Is phosphorylated tau unique to chronic traumatic encephalopathy? Phosphorylated tau in epileptic brain and chronic traumatic encephalopathy. Brain Res 2016;1630:225–40.

[134] Wen Y, Yang S, Liu R, Simpkins JW. Transient cerebral ischemia induces site-specific hyperphosphorylation of tau protein. Brain Res 2004;1022:30–8.

[135] Dewar D, Graham DI, Teasdale GM, McCulloch J. Cerebral ischemia induces alterations in tau and ubiquitin proteins. Dementia 1994;5:168–73.

[136] Hu HT, Xiao F, Yan YQ, Wen SQ, Zhang L. The prognostic value of serum tau in patients with intracerebral hemorrhage. Clin Biochem 2012;45:1320–4.

[137] Zanier ER, Longhi L, Fiorini M, et al. Increased levels of CSF heart-type fatty acid-binding protein and tau protein after aneurysmal subarachnoid hemorrhage. Acta Neurochir Suppl 2008;102:339–43.

[138] Julien JP, Mushynski WE. Neurofilaments in health and disease. Prog Nucleic Acid Res Mol Biol 1998;61:1–23.

[139] Buki A, Povlishock JT. All roads lead to disconnection? — Traumatic axonal injury revisited. Acta Neurochir (Wien) 2006;148:181–93; discussion 93–4.

[140] Zurek J, Bartlova L, Fedora M. Hyperphosphorylated neurofilament NF-H as a predictor of mortality after brain injury in children. Brain Inj 2012;25:221–6.

[141] Vajtr D, Benada O, Linzer P, et al. Immunohistochemistry and serum values of S-100B, glial fibrillary acidic protein, and hyperphosphorylated neurofilaments in brain injuries. Soud Lek 2013;57:7–12.

[142] Radwan W, El-Sabbagh A, Atweh S, Sawaya R. Ischaemic stroke with headache as its only manifestation. N Z Med J 2012;125:75–7.

[143] Sellner J, Patel A, Dassan P, Brown MM, Petzold A. Hyperacute detection of neurofilament heavy chain in serum following stroke: a transient sign. Neurochem Res 2011;36:2287–91.

[144] Singh P, Yan J, Hull R, et al. Levels of phosphorylated axonal neurofilament subunit H (pNfH) are increased in acute ischemic stroke. J Neurol Sci 2011;304:117–21.

[145] Nylen K, Csajbok LZ, Ost M, et al. CSF-neurofilament correlates with outcome after aneurysmal subarachnoid hemorrhage. Neurosci Lett 2006;404:132–6.

[146] Cai JY, Lu C, Chen MH, et al. Predictive value of phosphorylated axonal neurofilament subunit H for clinical outcome in patients with acute intracerebral hemorrhage. Clin Chim Acta 2013;424:182–6.

Chapter 8

Image-Guided Hypofractionated Radiosurgery of Large and Complex Brain Lesions

Dilini Pinnaduwage, Peng Dong and Lijun Ma

Additional information is available at the end of the chapter

http://dx.doi.org/10.5772/64481

Abstract

Hypofractionated radiosurgery either through frame or image guidance has emerged as the most important area of research and development for intracranial and extracranial radiosurgery. In this chapter, we focused on discussions of three state-of-the-art platforms: Frame- and Image-Guided Gamma Knife, Robotic X-Band Cykerknife, and Flattening-Filter-Free intensity-modulated S-band medical linear accelerators. Practical principles with detailed workflow and clinical implementations are presented in a systematic approach. With rapid evolvement of both hardware and software in the realm of delivering hypofractionated radiosurgery, this chapter aims to offer a reader physical clarity on judging and balancing of achieving high-precision and high-quality treatments with practical examples and guidelines on intracranial applications.

Keywords: hypofractionation, radiosurgery, Gamma Knife, Cyberknife, flattening filter free, linear accelerator

1. Hypofractionated Gamma Knife radiosurgery

The genesis of radiosurgery dated to the late 1940s when Swedish neurosurgeon Professor Dr. Lars Leksell pioneered the first stereotactic radiosurgery (SRS) device called Gamma Knife. The basic concept of radiosurgery (e.g., performing surgery without a scapel but with invisible photon rays) was revolutionary at the time, and it took several trials for Leksell to convince his peers and published his first paper on the device [1].

A key turning point in worldwide utilization of Gamma Knife radiosurgery (GKSRS) was its first North American installation at the University of Pittsburgh in 1987 [2]. Gradually and steadily, GKSRS has been demonstrated to be a highly successful modality in managing many benign and malignant indications [3–9]. However, due to the finite beam collimation size (maximum beam collimator diameter of 1.6–1.8 cm) and manual setups of individual patients, majority of the targets treated are relatively small lesions (e.g., <4 or 5 cm in maximum target dimension) and are generally treated in a single fraction [6, 9].

In 2006, GKSRS system underwent a redesign from ground up and the Leksell Gamma Knife Perfexion (PFX) was introduced in 2006, first in France, the UK, and then in the USA [10–13]. The key features of the PFX included an automatic submillimeter patient-positioning couch and a universal collimator system automatically aligns the radiation beamlets for variable collimation sizes. These new improvements physically eliminated manual setups of the early GKSRS models. As a result, GKSRS treatment delivery has become a turnkey solution and a large number of isocenters to be readily delivered with the minimum treatment effort. This greatly expanded the traditional GKSRS capability of treating large targets with a high number of isocenters.

With the advent of imaging guidance, the most recently developed Leksell Gamma Knife Icon (LGKI) has enabled repeatable patient setups without an invasive immobilization of an invasive metal frame, thus ushered in a new era of delivering hypofractionated GKSRS without number of isocenter restrictions. The general practice principles of GKSRS and its associated technical features of LGKI are described in detail in this section.

1.1. General physical principles

Unlike traditional C-arm radiation therapy delivery where a single source of radiation is employed and the radiation beams are delivered one beam after another in a sequential manner, GKSRS was designed from the start to employ hundreds of radiation beams to cross-fire in a simultaneous manner. In general, radiosurgical treatment delivery can be classified into four-type treatment delivery paradigms: (1) immobilize patient and radiation beams together, (2) mobilize patient and radiation beams together, (3) immobilize patient but mobilize radiation beams, and (4) mobilize patient but immobilize radiation beams.

The first and second types of treatment delivery are uncommon and employed primarily in specialized treatments such as ocular melanoma treatment, etc. Most of modern linac-based radiosurgical treatments employed the third type of delivery, where the patient or the treatment target was typically immobilized through various means, and radiation beams are delivered in sequence with the general assumption that patient's or target's position remained unchanged during the beam irradiation.

In contrast, GKSRS is a classic example of employing the fourth type of delivery, that is, all the radiation beams were fixed and the patient's positioning are adjusted from time to time to allow radiation dose delivered to different spots inside a 3D target volume. As a result, the overall precision involved in the treatment for GKSRS is largely governed by the positioning accuracy of the patient itself. The latest GKSRS PFX and Icon device have further improved general accuracy of GKSRS by employing fully digitally controlled patient positioning system (PPS) and patient surveillance system (PSS). With frame-based as well as latest infrared marker-based patient positioning monitoring capability, the system has been updated to detect mechanical shifts in the range of a few microns.

Figure 1 shows the latest GKSRS device, that is, the PFX and LGKI unit. Unlike previous GKSRS models, both PFX and LGKI employ a combination of the third and the fourth delivery paradigm as discussed above to achieve unmatched dose painting in the treatment planning process (the details of such a capability are described in the following section). In another word, once the patient is immobilized and aligned based on a pre-prescribed fixed position, the radiation beams become changeable while the patient is in position through a unique universal collimator system and a fully automatic couch patient positioning system as shown in the panel (a) of **Figure 1**. The details of the system components of the PFX and LGKI for hypofractionated GKSRS are described in the following paragraphs.

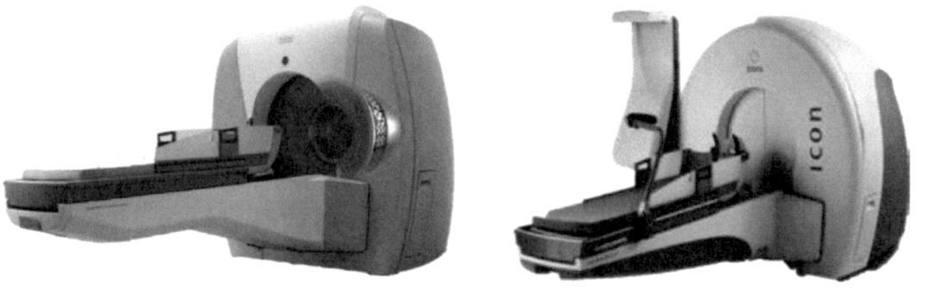

(a) (b)

Figure 1. (a) The Leksell Gamma Knife Perfexion (PFX) units and (b) Lekesell Gamma Knife Icon (LGKI) unit. Both systems possessed the same radiation generation mechanism through 192 Co-60 beams and a tungsten universal collimator behind a shield door as shown in Panel (a). The key difference between the two systems is the addition of a stereostatic cone-beam CT arm mounted for the LGKI unit as shown in Panel (b).

In summary, current GKSRS delivery through either PFX or LGI has enabled a combination of treatment delivery paradigms that successfully integrated mechanisms of precision patient immobilization (either with relocatable frame of PFX or with imaging-guided masking system of LGI) and the precision radiation beam alignment techniques to deliver adaptive hypofractional radiosurgical treatments. In the words of the Professor Dr. Lars Leksell, inventor of Gamma Knife: "The tools used by the surgeons must be adapted to the task and where the human brain is concerned they cannot be too refined". This is certainly the case for hypofractionated brain radiosurgery.

1.2. System design, hardware and work flow

One of the hallmarks of GKSRS was its Leksell G-frame system for immobilization of the skull of a patient. Besides being sturdy in securing and immobilizing the patient's skull for beam referencing, a major physical advantage of the frame is its elimination of rotational shifts required in patient setups. In another word, any point in the space can be readily reached with simple translational shifts along *x*-, *y*-, and *z*-directions once the frame has established its Cartesian coordinate system. However, due to invasive nature of the frame and current medical reimbursement rules in the USA, the frame-based GKSRS treatment was primarily limited to the single fraction GKSRS.

Recognizing the restrictions with the metal frame for delivering hypofractionated treatments, a vacuum-assisted relocatable frame system, that is, GK eXtend [14–17] was introduced shortly after the introduction of the PFX system in 2006. **Figure 2** illustrated the construction of such a relocatable frame system in actual clinical practice.

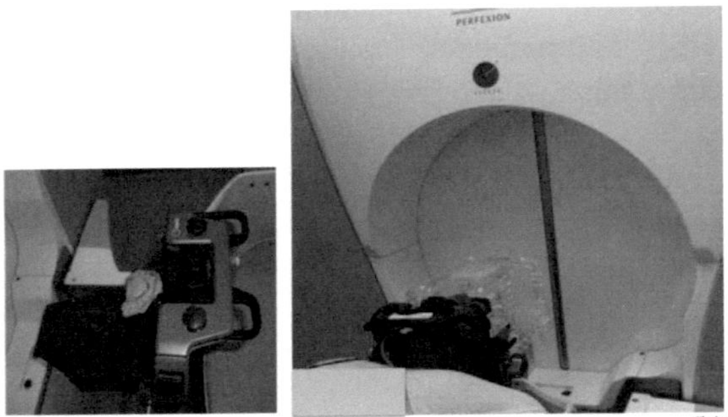

(a) (b)

Figure 2. Illustration of the GKSRS relocatable eXtend frame system shows: (a) the components of the customized eXtend frame with bite-block molded and docked onto the PFX unit and (b) the actual patient using the eXtend frame prior to the treatment delivery.

The relocatable frame as shown in the figure was adapted and improved over the conventional radiation therapy bite-block immobilization device. One major improvement is the use of vacuum assistance and saliva control cups that allow the bite-block to be anchored unto the hard palate in the patient's mouth. Together with vacuum cushion of the headrest (**Figure 3a**) supporting the back of the patient's skull, the patient's head immobilized with respect to the two lateral posts that is attached to the couch.

Evidently, the accuracy of such a relocatable frame depends on the positioning repeatability of the patient. **Figure 3b** shows the plastic template box attached to the superior of the patient head for such a purpose. The plastic template box was used to check the repeatability of the frame setup through the traditional dip-stick measurements, where the skull surface of variable points was measured before the treatment to ensure correct frame setups. In the case of eXtend frame showing in **Figure 3b**, such measurements were manually conducted through a calibrated digital probe, and measurement results were compared with the reference values taken at the time of the patient's CT scanning. An illustration of the probe measurement in conjunction with the patient setup of **Figure 2** is shown in **Figure 4**.

Several studies utilizing the PFX eXtend system have reported in-phantom as well as in-patient accuracy of 1 mm or less [16, 17]. One study primarily investigated the whole-procedural accuracy of the hypofractionated GKSRS treatments through the generalized end-to-end Winston-Lutz measurements as well as intrafractional patient data analysis [16]. The 3D radiological setup accuracy was determined to be 0.69 ± 0.73 mm (1σ) from a series of $n = 58$

http://dx.doi.org/10.5772/64481

treatment session, and the mean 90% confidence level range of uncertainties was found to be 0.55, 0.78, and 0.72 mm along the x-, y-, and z-axis, respectively.

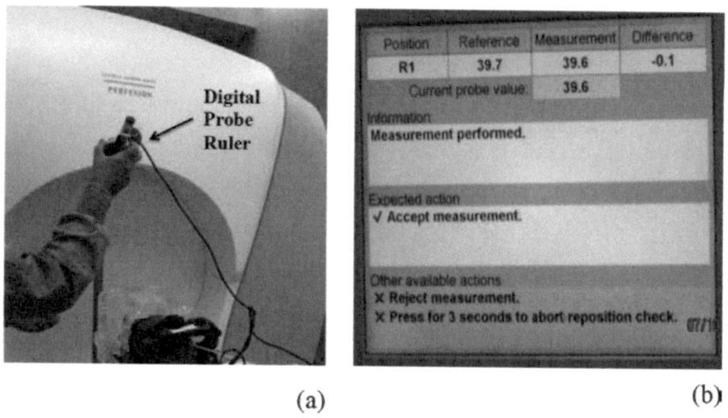

Figure 3. Illustration of the digital probe measurements for the hypofractionated GKSRS setups with the relocatable eXtend frame system on the PFX unit shows: (a) the hand-held digital probe ruler with the actual patient setups and (b) the measurement result of the probe at one template position. The difference displayed between the reference measurement and the actual measurement in (b) was in the unit of millimeter.

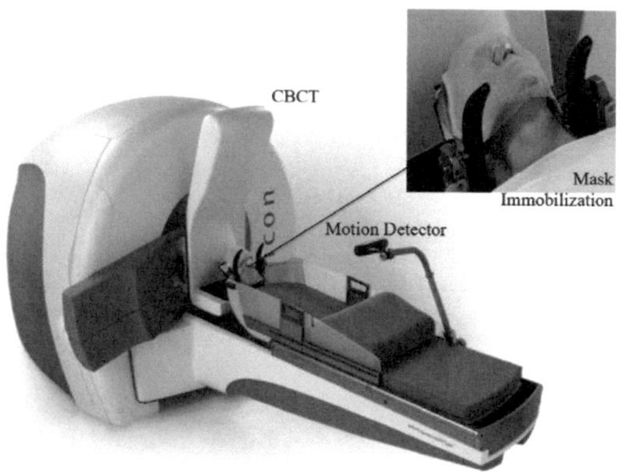

Figure 4. Major add-on system components of the Gamam Knife Icon (GKI) compared to the PFX include (1) a patient masking immobilization system (upper insert); (2) an on-line 3D imaging capability with stereotactic calibrated cone-beam CT device; and (3) a high-definition patient motion monitoring detector and feedback control system.

Evidently, the whole-procedural accuracy of these measurements included the positioning accuracy by the full couch motions. Given that multiple shots are typically used for hypofractionated treatments of relatively large lesions, the wear-and-tear of the couch in performing thousands of the patient setups may become a concern to ensure submillimeter accuracy. To investigate such problem, the central positioning as well as off-center couch positioning consistency was investigated through the so-called "picket fence" testing for a high-volume treatment center [18]. The study found an overall accuracy consistency of 0.03 ± 0.24 (2σ) mm. Such a value matched excellently with the manufacturer's mechanical specification of 0.35 mm even after repeated use of completing >1000 treatment cases. Based on the results of the study, the overall 3D vector accuracy was predominantly contributed by patient-specific rather than hardware-related in hypofractionated GKSRS treatments with the relocatable eXtend frame system.

Of note, patients to be treated with eXtend frame system need to be carefully selected before applying the relocatable eXtend frame system, specifically in regard to the performance status, gum health, and teeth integrity. With a team of experienced radiation therapy, users familiar with fabrication of conventional radiation therapy bite-blocks and managing patient's oral hygiene, hypofractionated GKSRS treatment with the PFX eXtend frame was an excellent option for expanding the traditional single-fractional GKSRS program.

Nearly a decade from the initial introduction of GK PFX system in 2006, US Food and Drug Administration and Nuclear Regulatory Commission have recently approved the image-guided Gamma Knife Icon (GKI) system. The GKI system is an integration of the PFX system with a 3D CBCT and a high-definition patient motion management system as shown in **Figure 5**. The 3D CBCT was designed to correct both translational and rotational shifts encountered during the initial patient setups when immobilized with the mask system. The patient motion management system monitors the patient's head positioning during the treatment delivery through a reflective marker placed on the patient's nose bridge in reference to the two lateral black post points as shown in the insert of **Figure 5**.

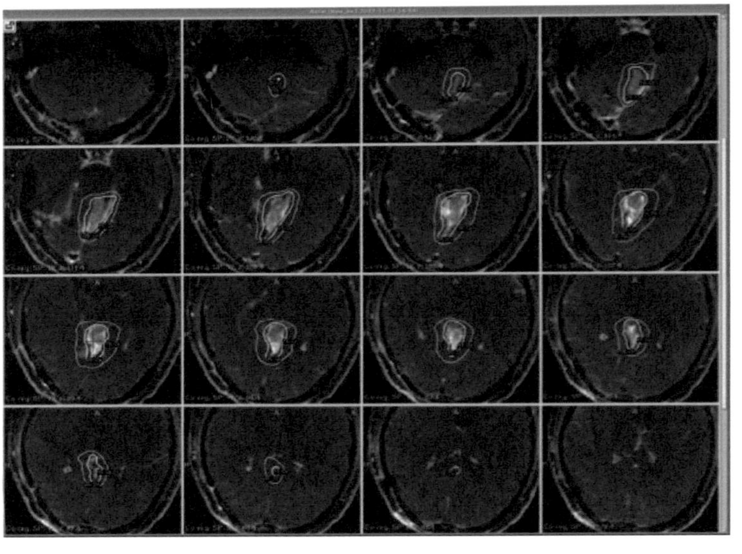

Figure 5. Axial dose distributions of a hypofractionated GKSRS treatment as planned with Leksell Gamma Plan (LGP version 10.2) for PFX or GKI treatments. Note the sharp dose fall-off along the posterior portion of the brainstem for maximum dose sparing.

The hypofractionated GKSRS workflow is similar among the eXtend frame system and the mask-based GKI system, where patient will undergo traditional MR and CT scans before the

http://dx.doi.org/10.5772/64481

treatment. However, the available of online 3D imaging guidance as offered by the GKI system allows the patient to be scanned without a tertiary frame, thus artifacts or susceptibility uncertainties introduced by these devices are eliminated from the workflow. In essence, on-device 3D CBCT serves not only as a "virtual" stereotactic frame but also as on-treatment patient positioning detection system.

Another important feature of GKI is its online dose recalculation and/or dose adaption workflow based on the 3D positioning as detected in vivo. In another word, once the patient position is measured by the CBCT, the 3D dose distribution based on the live patient setups (i.e., target location) will be recalculated and reference to the original treatment planning generated dose distributions. The attending physician and authorized medical physicist (AMP) for the treatment are afforded the opportunity to review or revise and approve the treatment plan before initiation of actual treatment delivery. The unique dose sculpting capability of the Leksell Gamma Plan (LGP) allows such a process to be an efficient and robust procedure.

1.3. Treatment planning and dosimetric evaluation

Compared to the early GKSRS treatment delivery, a user quickly would notice a major paradigm shift in planning PFX or GKI-based treatment delivery versus the previous Gamma Knife models. Traditionally, each isocenter or called a "shot" in the GKSRS is set and verified either manually or semi-manually through a tertiary add-on manipulator. As a result, using fewer numbers of shots to accomplish a treatment plan is desirable to ensure treatment delivery efficiency and patient comfort. Therefore, a user tends to optimize a treatment plan with mindset of minimizing the total number of shots as much as possible.

With the automatic full couch positioning system as in PFX or GKI, delivering multiple shots has become a turnkey solution. This has significantly shifted treatment-planning practices and in essence rendered hypofractionated treatment of relatively large or complex lesions a logical fit for planning with the PFX or GKI system. Without repeating many excellent reviews on classical GKSRS treatment planning techniques, we here focus on specific issues related to the hypofractionted treatment planning.

Figure 6 illustrated a 3D axial isodose distribution of a large hypofractionated GKSRS meningioma case, where 25 Gy in five fractions were prescribed to 50% of the maximum dose inside the target. Note the significant sharper dose fall-off along the brainstem surface area for the lesion as created by the planner when applying a relatively high number of shots ($n = 28$) and liberal use of the smallest collimator shots (i.e., 4 mm in nominal beam diameter) along the brainstem surface area.

Since single-session dose of 5 Gy is significantly lower than the traditional GKSRS of 15–20 Gy per session, the total number of shots can be used is therefore largely constrained by the minimum amount of radiation that can be delivered per shot. For example, if the maximum dose rate for the given treatment session is 3 Gy per minute, then 0.3 Gy would be minimum dose required per shot within the mechanical timer accuracy of 0.1 min per shot. As a result, the contribution from each shot should be at least 0.3 Gy for this case, thus limiting the total number of shots may be used for delivering such a treatment. This is a unique phenomenon for hypofractionated GKSRS.

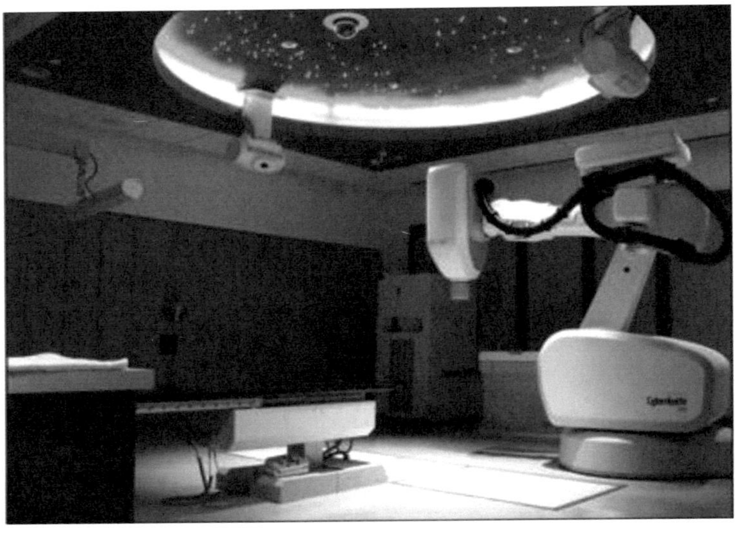

Figure 6. The Cyberknife VSI system installed in a clinical setting. Note the two X-ray tubes mounted on the ceiling and the X-ray detectors that are placed beneath the floor of the treatment vault for stereotactic imaging and on-line tracking.

Evaluation of hypofractionated GKSRS treatment plans as illustrated in **Figure 6** is identical to the conventional GKSR, that is, dosimetric treatment planning indices such as Paddick conformity index (PCI) [19] and gradient index (GI) [20] similarly apply to single as well as hypofractionated GKSRS.

In summary, the PCI is defined as $PCI = (TIV)^2/(PIV \times TV)$, where TIV is the volume of the target falls inside 100% of the prescription isodose surface, PIV is the total 100% prescription isodose volume, and TV is the total target volume. In parallel, the GI is defined as $GI = PIV50/PIV$, where PIV50 is the total isodose volume enclosed by 50% of the prescription dose.

From the definitions of PCI and GI of the above, PCI is a direct measurement of how well the prescription isodose volume match or "conform" to the target volume, and GI is the measure of how steep the planned dose distribution falls beyond the prescription isodose surface. Studies have been carried out to investigate the best possible dose gradient that can be achieved for general GKSRS, and an empirical power law was found to describe such a dose fall-off near perfectly yielding high linear correlation of > 90% [12, 21].

In the context of hypofractionated treatment delivery, it is worth noting that PIV50 can be easily replaced with PIV30, PIV40, PIV60, etc. (e.g., 30, 40, 60, etc.) prescription isodose volumes to expand the definition of GI and allow detailed survey of the isodose dose effects associated with hypofractionated treatments. Unlike single fractional GKSRS delivery where peripheral isodose volumes around PIV50 such as the 10-Gy or 12-Gy isodose volumes have been reported

http://dx.doi.org/10.5772/64481

to surrogated the treatment complications such as symptomatic radiation necrosis rate, relevant isodose volumes for variable fractionation schemes such as 3–5 fractions have yet been established. Therefore, a user need to be careful in examining the peripheral isodose fall-off measures such as the PIV30, PIV40 or PIV60, etc. for all treatments until future clinical data and guidelines become available.

1.4. Future direction and developments

With the advent of GKI, hypofractionated GKSRS treatments expected to expand rapidly in the years ahead. Initial studies have shown excellent precision as well as robustness for patient positioning correction capability that rival frame-based treatment deliveries. With reduced dose for each hypofractionated treatment session such as 5–8 Gy and integrated stereo-CBCT treatment setups with direct coordinates adaption, the overall treatment delivery time with GKI would be expected to be 30 min or less that making it match well with other treatment modalities.

Several studies have indicated superior dose sculpting capabilities of PFX and GKI versus early GK SRS models [11]. Further treatment planning studies have also suggested equivalency of linac-based delivery with an early GK model [22]. Such a result supports the general finding of superiority of PFX and GI versus the linac-based treatment in sparing normal brain tissues [23–25]. These studies have clearly fortified the leading role of GKSRS in performing intracranial hypofractionated SRS.

However, it is worth mentioning several ongoing efforts in continually improving the dosimetric capabilities of GKSRS. One study has proposed the notion of dynamic GKSR delivery, where the whole treatment can be delivered through single path motion (i.e., the beam is always on during a treatment) in contrast to the step-and-shoot type of delivery [26]. One major improvement in the dosimetric properties noted was the significant improvements in the dose homogeneity within the target as well as some improvements in the peripheral dose fall-off, a likely contribution from the increased number of the beams associated with the treatment delivery.

Another study leveraging the power of sector beam mixing has proposed the concept of simultaneous intensity modulation for GKSRS [27]. In the mode of such a delivery, the intensity levels in 2π arrangement become fully variable from either zero (closed sector beam) to unity (open sector beam) during each shot delivery. It was found that significant normal tissue sparing improvements achieved by adding the sector intensity modulation for complex treatment cases such as epilepsy and for large lesion treatments involving a high number of isocenters. The latter of which is clearly relevant for the hypofractionated GKSRS. One key advantage noted with sector-beam intensity modulation is that the total beam-on time is equivalent to the traditional nonmodulated treatment deliveries thus making the approach clinically ready with the current PFX and GKI hardware design. Ongoing and further studies will determine whether dosimetric improvements as discussed above would translate into clear clinical advantages, especially in the developments of hypofractionated GKSRS.

2. Hypofractionated robotic CyberKnife radiosurgery

The CyberKnife (CK) is an image-guided, frameless, robotic radiosurgery system invented by John Adler and his team in the late 1980s [28, 29]. Unlike in the Gamma Knife system where Gamma rays from Co-60 decay are used for treatments, the CyberKnife system uses X-rays generated from a linear accelerator for radiation treatments. While the system received FDA clearance to treat head and neck, and upper spine lesions in 1999, in 2001, clearance was given to treat lesions located anywhere in the body. Therefore, the current system can be used for both intracranial and extracranial (spine, lung, liver, pelvis, etc.) radiation treatments. The CK system is not only an integrated unit consisting of treatment planning, imaging, and delivery, but also unique in its ability to continuously track, detect, and correct for both tumor and patient motion during treatment.

2.1. System descriptions and working principle

CyberKnife treatments are delivered through a motorized robotic manipulator (KUKA robot) that is attached to a lightweight X-band linear accelerator (linac) (**Figure 3**). The robotic manipulator allows for six degrees of freedom in positioning the radiation source, and allows for noncoplanar, nonisocentric beam delivery. The linac generates 6 MV photons, at a nominal dose rate of up to 1000 cGy/min. The manipulator is programmed to move within a fixed, predetermined workspace, and positions the radiation source at pre-assigned points within this workspace referred to as "nodes". At each node, the linac can deliver radiation from multiple beam angles [30]. Dose is delivered from "paths," which comprise of a series of nodes, determined during treatment planning. During treatment delivery, the manipulator moves the accelerator from node to node in sequence and delivers dose at those nodes selected during planning. The treatment path adopted by the robotic manipulator is dependent on the target location and patient anatomy as specified during treatment planning.

The radiation is collimated using either 12 interchangeable tungsten cones (known as "fixed" collimators), or the Iris™ (a variable aperture collimator [31]), both with aperture diameters ranging from 5 to 60 mm at a SAD of 800 mm. The Iris™ is made of two offset banks of six tungsten segments each, which combine to create dodecahedral apertures. With the Iris, the robot traverses the treatment path only once while delivering radiation from multiple collimating apertures at the chosen node position. In comparison, with the CK fixed cone system, the robot has to traverse the treatment path separately for each fixed cone size used for the treatment. Therefore, the Iris allows the use of multiple collimating apertures for a given treatment without drastically increasing treatment time. The newly released CK M6 platform, available for clinical use today, is additionally equipped with a multi leaf collimating (MLC) system that provides further potential for improved efficiency in the treatment delivery. This MLC system (CK InCise MLC system, Accuray Inc.) consists of 41 tungsten leaf pairs of 90 mm height and 2.5mm thickness at 800 mm SAD, and allows for a maximum field size of 120 (in the leaf motion direction) × 100 mm at 800 mm SAD. Leaf motion allows for 100% over-travel and full leaf inter-digitation, and has an average (intra-leaf, inter-leaf, and leaf tip) transmission of <0.3% [32].

The tracking volume (or the target volume itself) is stereotactically localized using orthogonal kV X-ray images. X-rays in the diagnostic energy range are generated from two X-ray sources that are attached to the treatment room ceiling. The X-rays exiting the patient are detected by amorphous silicon flat panel detectors, which are embedded beneath the floor. The imaging center, or the point in space at which these imaging beams intersect, is referred to as the "align center". The geometry of the imaging system is such that the patient is imaged at a 45° angle. The high-resolution digital X-ray images obtained during patient setup and treatment are automatically registered to a set of digitally reconstructed radiographs (DRRs) generated from the treatment planning CT. The difference in patient positioning from simulation to treatment in the three translation and rotational directions are calculated based on this 2D–2D registration. During treatment, the patient is imaged at an imaging frequency that can be specified by the operator. The imaging frequency can be set between 15 and 150 sec, and it is common to image the patient at time intervals of 30–60 sec in the case of brain treatments. During treatment delivery, the robotic manipulator compensates for the differences seen in the patient, or target position, by redirecting the radiation beam to the actual target position in near-real time.

2.2. Treatment simulation and inverse planning

Proper patient simulation is critical to ensure an accurate treatment delivery. While it is imperative in radiation therapy in general, to achieve a patient setup that is both easily reproducible and comfortable for the patient, for CK treatments the patient setup should in addition adhere to specific patient safety zone requirements. The CK system consists of two virtual safety zones, named the "fixed safety zone" and the "dynamic safety zone". These safety zones are designed as safety mechanisms to prevent robot collisions with the patient. The fixed safety zone is based on the imaging center and varies in dimension depending on the treatment site (i.e., head vs. body). The dynamic safety zone is located within the fixed safety zone [30, 33]. It includes all of the patient body and varies in size based on the individual patient's size (small, medium, and large) as specified by the therapist.

For brain treatments, custom-made head masks are used to immobilize the patient. An appropriate headrest is chosen so that the patient's neck is in a comfortable position. In particular, hyperextended or flexed neck positions are discouraged, as treatment times can be as long as 30 min for a typical brain treatment. The treatment times could be even longer for multiple brain metastasis treatments, based on the number of lesions, lesion size, and prescription dose to each. The patient's arms and knees should be placed in compliance with the patient safety zone requirements discussed above.

CT simulation is performed with the patient in the supine position. A contiguous, no gap CT scan is obtained with a 1–1.5 mm slice thickness. The slice thickness is important as thinner slices generate better quality DRRs improving the tracking accuracy [34]. The CT field-of-view should be reasonable (typically 30 cm) and not unnecessarily large for improved image quality. The scan should be centered on the target and includes the entire patient head as the tracking algorithm for brain treatments is based on the patient's skull features. The primary CT used for treatment planning should be a noncontrast CT as contrast in the scan may impact dose calculation and tracking accuracy. If a contrast CT is needed, the contrast CT can be imported into the planning system as a secondary image set.

2.2.1. *Image registration and structure contouring*

For brain CK treatments, MR imaging is used for target delineation because MR provides better soft tissue visualization compared to CT. Certain critical structures such as the brainstem and chiasm are also better visualized on MR. Because dose calculation for treatment planning is based on CT, the MR images are imported into the planning system as secondary image set and coregistered with the primary CT data set. Several image registration options are available within the CK treatment planning software. For most brain cases, the automatic registration feature is commonly used, and the user can specify the region of interest for the auto-registration. This algorithm uses intensity values based on mutual information. In addition, a semiautomatic point based, and manual registration methods are also available. Once target contouring is complete, critical structures are delineated. MR images are then used to define certain critical structures such as the brainstem and chiasm, whereas the some other structures such as the optic nerves and cochlea can be better defined based on the planning CT.

The difficulty level of treatment planning for brain lesions can vary depending on the target location and proximity to critical structures such as the brain stem and optic structures. For those cases in which the critical structures are in close proximity to the target volume, planning risk volumes (PRVs) may be generated by expanding those critical structures by ~2–3 mm and by ensuring that these PRV volumes are well within their dose tolerance during the treatment planning process. Another option is to generate a new planning target volume (PTV) by subtracting the expanded critical structure from the original PTV. The treatment plan can then be optimized using this "modified PTV" to confine the portion of the PTV receiving less than the prescription dose to the PTV-critical structure interface. By targeting the radiation beams to the edges of the "modified PTV" instead of the original PTV by applying beam collimators to the modified PTV, a sharper dose gradient can be created at the PTV-critical structure interface, allowing for better sparing of the critical structure while maintaining good dose coverage of the target volume. The collimator size chosen for beam generation is dependent on the target dimensions, complexity and location. Either the fixed or the Iris™ collimating systems can be used. However, with the fixed cones, the number of cone sizes is typically limited to three to reduce treatment time, because as mentioned previously in this chapter during treatment delivery, the robot has to traverse the treatment path with each cone separately. This limitation in the number of aperture diameters to be selected is not a concern when using the Iris™, as the robot can change apertures at a given beam position during single treatment path traversal. The smallest Iris™ apertures (i.e., 5 and 7.5 mm) are typically avoided during treatment planning as small differences in field size can result in significantly large differences in beam output [35, 36].

Once the user selects the beam apertures, a set of a few thousand-candidate beams is generated. These beams are defined based on the node positions, target location, and collimators chosen. Either isocentric targeting or conformal targeting can be chosen for planning CK brain cases. In isocentric targeting, all beams point toward a single user specified target location within the

http://dx.doi.org/10.5772/64481

tumor, and there is only one beam per node position. Isocentric planning is mostly used for simple cases, where the lesion is nearly spherical and not adjacent to critical structures. With conformal targeting, beams target multiple locations within the tumor. The target points are randomly distributed over the tumor perimeter, and multiple beams per node position are utilized. A typical plan consists of over a hundred nonisocentric, noncoplanar beams (**Figure 7b**) in the conformal targeting scenario. Conformal targeting is useful for complicated brain cases. Beam entry through the eyes is typically prohibited.

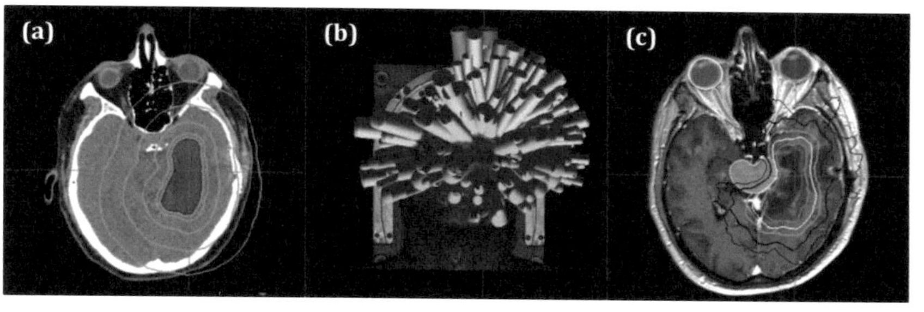

Figure 7. (a) Shell structures (a total of five shown here) generated surrounding the planning target volume to improve dose conformity and produce sharp dose gradients outside of the target. (b) A 3D representation of the beam angles used for an example CK brain treatment in which over a hundred nonisocentric, noncoplanar beams are being used. (c) Isodose distribution for an example CK brain treatment in which the planning target volume abuts the brain stem. The dose distribution is displayed on the MR images used for target delineation.

The user can also constrain the total number of monitor units (MUs) to be used for a plan, as well as specify the monitor units that should be used per node and per beam. Constraining the contribution of monitor units (MUs) from a given beam/node allows a wider distribution (or spread in beam angles) of nonisocentric, noncoplanar beams, and limits a high dose contribution from a single direction. This helps minimize "dose fingers" (high dose (typically >40–50% of the prescription dose) streaks/areas spanning from outside of the target volume toward the skin, that are shaped similar to a finger) and dose hot spots in normal tissue. The maximum MUs per node were set to be slightly higher than the maximum MUs per beam to allow for multiple beams per node. For a typical brain plan, the total MUs are ~5–10 times the prescription dose.

The dose distribution is optimized by adjusting the weighting of the beam MUs in the candidate beam set generated based on the user specified dose objectives/constraints, to minimize a linear cost function. Sequential optimization [37] is commonly used in treatment planning, where different optimization objectives such as target coverage, conformity, and dose constraints to critical structures are addressed sequentially in a user-specified order. The optimization moves from one step to the next, only when those goals set by the planner are met within user-specified relaxation criteria. This allows the user to prioritize goals (i.e., target coverage vs. critical structure sparing) in a clinically significant patient specific manner. MultiPlan^{TM} (the CyberKnife treatment planning software) further allows for the generation of multiple shell structures of varying radii surrounding the target volume (**Figure 7a**). Dose constraints applied to these shells can be manipulated to achieve a highly conformal plan and to guide and tighten the dose fall of outside of the target volume. In addition, beam reduction and time reduction tools are available to the planner to assess and improve plan efficiency without compromising plan quality.

The CK treatment planning system provides two dose calculation algorithms: (1) Ray-tracing and (2) Monte Carlo. Ray-tracing uses the effective path length to determine dose deposition based on tissue heterogeneities, and is based on a pencil beam approach in which a single beam is considered to constitute of many single rays [33]. However, photon scatter and lateral electron scatter in heterogeneous media are not correctly accounted for with Ray-tracking as is with Monte Carlo. This results in substantial inaccuracies in dose calculation at the interface of tissues of different densities and for those lesions that are located within low-density (i.e., lung, sinuses) and high-density (i.e., bone) tissues [38]. For example, for lung cases, using Ray-tracing for dose calculation can result in 8–11% differences compared to that calculated with Monte Carlo [38]. For brain lesions that are not adjacent to, or in, air/bone, the differences in the plans calculated using Ray-tracing compared to Monte Carlo are clinically insignificant, with the differences in maximum dose to the critical structures and tumor coverage generally found to be <5% between the two calculation methods [39]. However, for those lesions that are located in/adjacent to the sinus cavity or bony anatomy, dose calculation with Monte Carlo may provide more accurate results. The Monte Carlo algorithm uses theoretical simulation and experimental results to calculate dose deposition from each particle traveling through tissue, considering its interactions with other particles. The Monte Carlo platform specifically employed within the CK treatment planning system uses a single source model, which simulates photon interactions with media for a variety of photon energies. The travel paths of the secondary electrons generated by the interaction of photons with tissue are further considered. Dose deposition by these charged particles is calculated considering tissue density differences and electron stopping powers [38].

2.2.2. *Typical treatment planning dose volume constraints*

Typical fractionation schemes for CK brain treatments are 25 or 30 Gy in five fractions. Single and three fraction dose schemes are also sometimes used. Dose constraints to critical structures are mainly based on those recommend by AAPMs Task Group Report [40] as given in **Table 1**.

		Single fraction		Three fractions		Five fractions	
Serial structure	**Max critical volume above threshold**	**Threshold dose (Gy)**	**Max point dose (Gy)**	**Threshold dose (Gy)**	**Max point dose (Gy)**	**Threshold dose (Gy)**	**Max point dose (Gy)**
Optic pathway	<0.2 cc	8	10	15.3	17.4	23	25
Cochlea			9		17.1		25
Brainstem (not medulla)	<0.5 cc	10	15	18	23.1	23	31
Spinal cord and medulla	<0.35 cc	10	14	18	21.9	23	30
	<1.2 cc	7		12.3		14.5	

Table 1. Dose constraints for hypofractionated brain treatments as recommended by AAPMs Task Group 101.

http://dx.doi.org/10.5772/64481

Figure 7c shows an example of a complicated brain CK plan in which the target volume abuts the brainstem. A prescription dose of 25 Gy was prescribed to the planning target volume in five fractions in this particular case. Dose was prescribed to the 70% isodose line. The brain stem maximum dose (0.035 cc) for this particular case was kept below 22 Gy. The optic chiasm maximum dose was <9 Gy and the optic nerve maximum dose was ~10 Gy. The gradient index and the conformality index (nCI) for this particular plan was 2.92 and 1.13, respectively. The dose distribution within the target volume is highly heterogeneous as is commonly the case for CK plans, because typical prescription isodose lines for brain treatments vary between 60 and 75%. However, with the CyberKnife, the planner can guide the optimization to achieve a plan prescribing to a wide range of isodoselines. Therefore, CK plans can be tailored to achieve plans similar to Gamma Knife plans (by optimizing the plan such that the prescription isodose is ~50%) or linac based SRS/SBRT plans (by optimizing the plan such that the prescription isodose is between 70 and 80%).

2.3. Clinical studies – hypofractionated brain treatments

Several clinical investigations have reported on the safety and efficacy of hypofractionated CK brain treatments. One such study [41] looking at CK treatments for large brain metastases delivering 30–41 Gy in 3–5 fractions, reported a crude local tumor control (LTC) rate of 86.8%. The estimated LTC rates at 12 and 24 months were 87 and 65.2%. The median overall survival and progression-free survival rates were 16 and 11 months, respectively. Patient performance status and preoperative neurologic deficits reportedly improved in 57.1 and 70.6%, respectively. Another study [42] evaluating the efficacy and toxicity of 5-fraction CK radiotherapy in patients with large brain metastases in critical areas, demonstrated that a high rate of local tumor control and low rate of complications are achievable. They report a local tumor control rate of 92.9% during a median follow-up of 8 months and report that neurological manifestations improved in 50.9% of the patients.

2.4. Intrafractional monitoring and treatment delivery

A 6D Skull Tracking is the tracking method used for CK brain treatments. This method is frameless and uses the bony anatomy of the skull obtained from 2D X-ray imaging for patient set up and for determining and correcting for patient motion during treatment delivery. This tracking method can be used for intracranial, head and neck, and certain upper spine (C1, C2) treatments. The algorithm assumes a fixed relationship, between the target, the "align center" and the bony anatomy of the skull. The "align center" (also referred to as the imaging center) is user defined during treatment planning. For brain treatments, the "align center" is chosen such that the superior and anterior parts of the skull are ~10–15 mm from the edge of the imaging field-of-view (**Figure 8**).

Prior to treatment start, the patient is immobilized and positioned as during simulation. Patient setup is carried out through a motorized couch, which has either 5 (standard couch) or 6 (RoboCouch^{TM}) degrees of freedom. A pair of X-ray images is taken to make gross adjustments to the patient position, which can then be fine-tuned using automatic couch movements. Correct positioning is confirmed by comparing the live X-ray images to DRRs from the treatment planning CT. The algorithm correlates the live X-ray images with the DRRs based on pixel similarity criteria. X-ray technique (kV, mAs and exposure time) needs to be optimized by using parameters provided by the software showing differences in the estimated align center position based on each image along the common superior/inferior axis, similarity of overall image intensity between the live images and the DRRs, and the presence of external objects in the X-ray image that are not on the DRR.

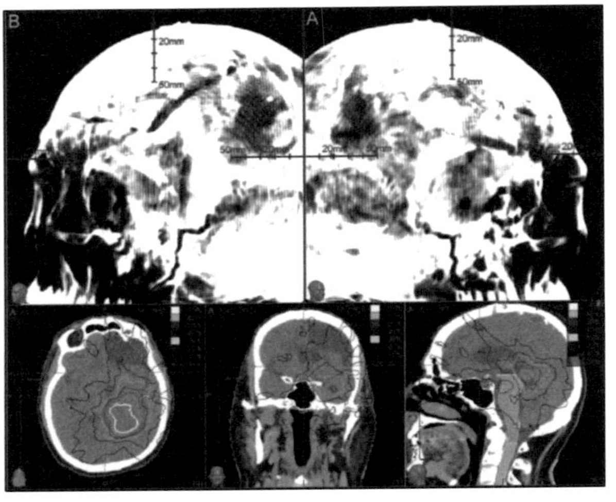

Figure 8. An example of how the "align center" or the imaging center is specified during treatment planning for an example CK brain treatment. The "align center" is chosen such that the superior and anterior parts of the skull on the DRRs are ~10–15 mm from the edge of the imaging field-of-view. The bottom portion displays the placement of the cross hairs on the planning CT images to achieve the appropriate placement of the skull on the DRR images as shown on the top panel.

Once the beam is on for treatment, orthogonal X-rays are intermittently taken (at time intervals of 30–60 sec (lower imaging interval can be chosen on a case-by-case basis). These images are automatically registered to the DRRs derived from the treatment planning CT. Unique to the CKS, the robotic manipulator uses this near real-time target position information to retarget the radiation beam to the current target position, thus eliminating the need for patient repositioning. The robot can automatically correct for translations up to 10 mm, and rotations of 1, 1, and 3° for the roll, yaw and pitch, respectively.

Submillimeter accuracy is achievable through 6D Skull Tracking. A recent study [43] used log files generated by the CKS, as well as the actual treatment parameters from each procedure to investigate the mechanical uncertainty in beam localization over a time period of approximately 1 year. They further evaluated patterns of patient movement during brain CK treatments. They found the mean mechanical uncertainties of CK brain tumor treatments to be 0.07, 0.01, and −0.09 mm in the +inferior/−superior, +left/−right, and +anterior/−posterior directions, respectively and conclude the CK to be robust in tracking accuracy regardless of patient's movement. Their investigations further found a CTV-PTV margin of 2.0 mm to be adequate in brain tumor treatments for an on-treatment imaging interval of 30–45 sec.

http://dx.doi.org/10.5772/64481

2.5. Future developments

As mentioned earlier in the chapter, a new CK system equipped with three interchangeable collimating systems (fixed, Iris, and MLC) is now available for clinical use. This new CK M6 platform has the potential to improve the efficiency of hypofractionated CK treatments and to further extend the advantages of noncoplanar treatment and real-time tracking to conventionally fractionated treatment. A recent study [44] assessing the clinical capabilities of the CK-MLC for hypofractionated brain SBRT demonstrated that treatment plans generated with the CK-MLC were of equal or better quality compared to clinically approved CK plans using circular (fixed/Iris™) collimators. The total monitor units were reduced by 70%, and the treatment time could be reduced by nearly a half by using the CK-MLC, with an average treatment time of 17 min compared to 30 min for plans using circular apertures.

3. Hypofractionated S-Band linac-based radiosurgery

In the 1986, Lutz and Winston described "A small field irradiation technique to deliver high doses of single fraction photon radiation to small, precisely located volumes (0.5–8 cm^3) within the brain". This marked the beginning of brain SRS with linear accelerators [45, 46]. Now 30 years later, the clinicians have a new generation of radiation therapy machines, which are designed from the ground up to combine the fast delivery of high dose rate from flattening filter free (FFF) beam and precise tumor localization with image guided radiotherapy (IGRT), at their service to push the boundary of SRS with escalated dose protocols and innovative fraction scheme, limiting side effects and sparing nearby organs at risk. **Figure 9** shows the two modern linear accelerators from Varian (left panel) and Elekta (right panel), respectively.

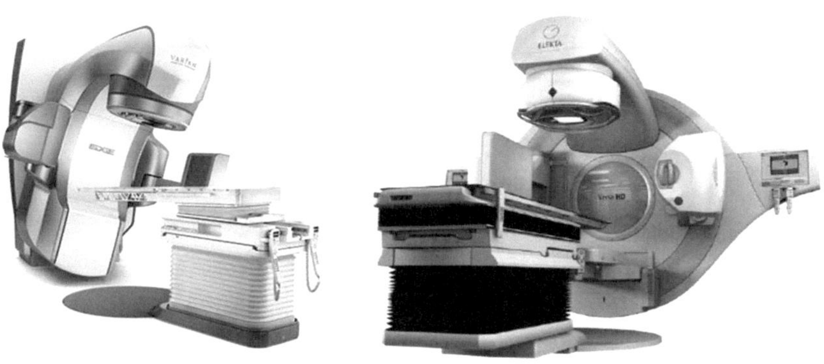

Figure 9. Two state-of-the-art medical linear accelerators that are capability of high-precision hypofractionated treatments: left panel shows Edge manufactured from Varian Oncology (Palo Alto, CA) and right panel shows Versa HD manufactured from Elekta Company (Atlanta, GA).

The newest generation of Linac from Varian, Edge, has X-ray output energies at 6MV (600 MU/min), 6X FFF mode (1400 MU/min) and 10X FFF mode (2400 MU/min). With gantry and collimator isocenters accuracy smaller than 0.5 mm radius, gantry, collimator, and couch isocenters accuracy smaller than 0.75 mm radius and gantry rotational accuracy smaller than 0.3°, the Edge has the mechanical performance required for SRS. The high definition 120 leaf MLC, moving at a maximum speed of 2.5 cm/sec, with an extra fine MLC leaf at 2.5 mm in the central 20 cm and 40 × 22 cm field size, can treat most of the smaller brain tumors.

Versa HD, the latest offering from Elekta, can treat patient with 6 MV-15 MV at 600 MU/min, 6× FFF mode at 1400 MU/min and 10× FFF mode at 2200 MU/min. It also carries the Agility MLC with 80 MLC pairs at 5 mm width across the full 40 × 40 cm field and a speed up to 3.5 cm/sec. When coupled with dynamic leaf guide, the MLC leaf move at an effective speed of 6.5 cm/sec. Gantry, collimator, and couch isocentricity measurements were within 1, 0.7, and 0.7 mm diameter, respectively [47].

3.1. Beam and patient positioning characteristics

3.1.1. Fast delivery with FFF beam and VMAT

The major drawback of performing SRS with a conventional linear accelerator is the long delivery time results from the low dose rate. For hypofractionated SRS with 2000 MU per fraction, the beam on time alone is ~3 min for conventional beams. In 1991, O'Brien PF presented in his paper that after removed the flattening filter from an AECL Therac-6 linear accelerator, the dose rate is increased by a factor of 2.75. Now almost all major linacs can operate in the FFF mode with maximum dose at ~2400 MU/min. Volumetric-modulated arc therapy, a rotational arc therapy with intensity modulation, achieves highly conformal dose distributions with great treatment delivery efficiency and reduced total MU. The VMAT delivery, in conjunction with the FFF mode, can lead to even greater efficiency in delivery. One study [48] compared VMAT FFF plan with IMRT flat beams and found that the mean beam-on time difference was 6.79 min (74.9% decrease); mean treatment delivery time difference was 8.99 min (range: 5.40–13.05 min), a relative improvement of 71.1% (range: 53.4–82.4%) for plans with high dose fractionations (16–20 Gy/fraction).

3.1.2. Patient positioning with frameless system

With the introduction of on board KV MV imaging and the development of image guided radiotherapy, frameless intracranial systems become an alternative to the invasive frames used traditionally to establish the stereotactic coordinates of the targets and ensure the accuracy of immobilization and positioning such as the Leksell stereotactic frame. The frameless SRS brings patient convenience and comfort, enables an efficient workflow for hypofractionation, and makes SRS more available where there is no neurosurgical support. **Figure 10** shows the Leksell frame, Brainlab frameless mask, and Civco's trUpoint Arch system.

The patient immobilization is ensured by the bite-block and thermoplastic masks. The six optical marking spheres on top of the Brainlab mask monitored by infrared camera on roof provide real-time tracking of the departure from the treatment isocenter and information to determine X-ray imaging frequency. One study has compared four frameless, thermoplastic mask-based immobilization strategies for inter- and intrafraction patient positioning uncertainties [49]. They studied four systems including: (1) head mask with head cushion; (2) head mask with head cushion and a body immobilizer; (3) head mask and cushion with shoulder mask and cushion; and (4) same as (3) plus a mouthpiece. The system (4) has a mean interfraction translational shift of 2.1 (±1.0) mm and intrafraction motion of 0.7 (±0.8) mm, providing the best accuracy and stability overall.

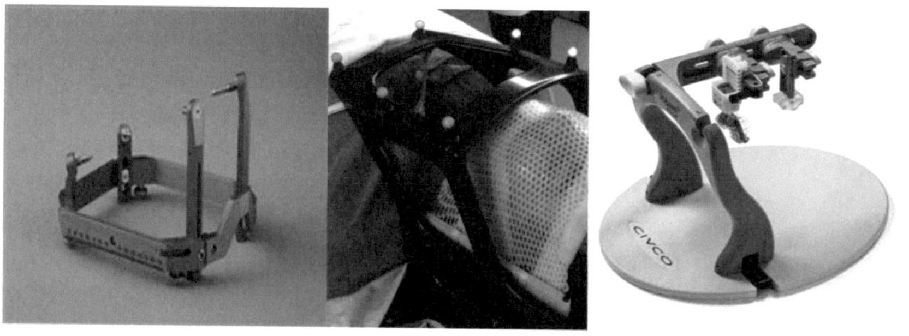

Figure 10. Left: Leksell frame; middle: Brainlab localization array mask; and right: CIVCO mask.

3.2. Imaging guidance

3.2.1. In-room KV/MV imaging

The comparison of the portal images from electronic portal imaging devices (EPID) with DRR is the most commonly used patient positioning verification, which can be performed with either KV on board imager providing higher soft tissue contrast or MV imaging with the treatment beam when bones or fiducial marks can be used for alignment. Usually an orthogonal image pair is acquired and followed by the automatic shift calculation with the computer and appropriate correction by the treatment couch. For an improvement of the target visualization, CBCT can also be performed. As a complementary to the on-linac imaging mainly for patient initial setup, several commercial product provide intrafraction continuous monitoring of the patient's position. The Exac-trac X-ray system consists of two oblique X-ray imagers, with two floor mounted KV X-ray tubes and two corresponding flat panel detectors on the ceiling (**Figure 11**). The system can take images at any gantry or couch angle. With the 6D fusion option, the system can calculate patient's position variation in three translational direction and three rotational directions. Another system to monitor intrafraction movement is through monitoring patient's surface features such as the AlignRt system, where a high-resolution 3D-rendered surface of the patient from the pseudo-random pattern projected on the patient's skin, using stereo vision techniques and a triangulation process without any ionization radiation.

3.2.2. Six degrees-of-freedom couch

With all the advancements of the field of IGRT, a further improvement of patient setup can be achieved by the new generation of six degrees-of-freedom (6DoF) couch that can correct the patient setup in three translational axes and three rotation axes. One group of investigators performed tests to request a known shift for the 6DoF couch and compared this requested shift with the actually applied shift by independently measuring the applied shift using different methods (graph paper, laser, inclinometer, and imaging system) [50]. The study found that the deviations were −0.01 ± 0.02, 0.01 ± 0.02, and 0.01 ± 0.02 cm for the longitudinal, lateral, and vertical axes, respectively; 0.03 ± 0.06, −0.04 ± 0.12, and −0.01 ± 0.08° for the three rotational axes couch rotation, pitch, and roll, respectively.

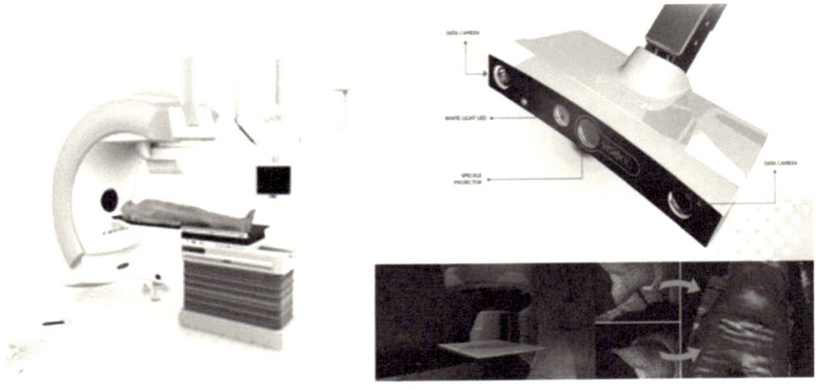

Figure 11. Left panel: Exactrac X-ray imaging system (Novalis) and right panel: surface-based patient alignment system (AlignRt).

The combination of in-room imaging and robotic couch can achieve high precision in cranial treatment of immobilized patients. One European group has demonstrated translational repositioning accuracy of 0.9 ± 0.5 mm for 47 consecutive patients with 372 fractions [51].

3.3. Treatment planning

3.3.1. Cone-based planning

By using cone collimators and multiple intersecting noncoplanar arcs, the linac can deliver dose distribution similar to that of the Gamma Knife. It produced a tight spherically shaped high dose region with sharp dose fall-off (**Figure 12**).

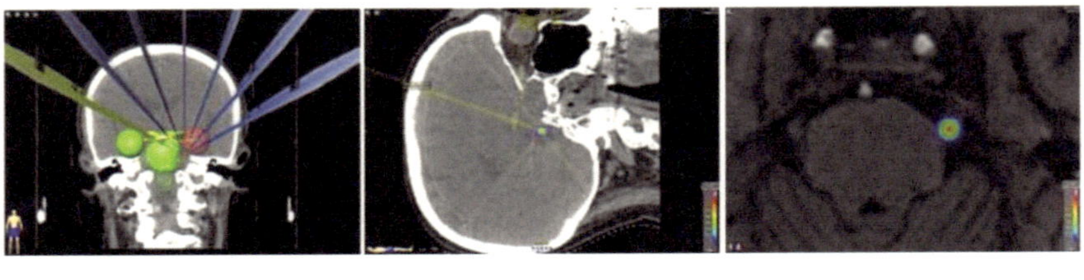

Figure 12. Illustration of a treatment plan case on the Brainlab system.

http://dx.doi.org/10.5772/64481

3.3.2. VMAT

VMAT offers shorter treatment times that are consistent with the goals of IGRT. It facilitates sparing proximal normal tissues compared to the fixed aperture techniques and simultaneously treating multiple targets with a single isocenter. One group showed that SRS using VMAT is a viable alternative to other techniques and enables short treatment times [52]. Another group replanned older model Gamma Knife (GK Model C) treatments of multiple cranial metastases with multi-arc (MA) and single-arc (SA), single-isocenter VMAT (RapidArc) in Eclipse [22]. They found that for multiple target SRS, 4-arc VMAT produced clinically equivalent conformity, dose fall-off, 12 Gy isodose volume, and low isodose spill, and reduced treatment time compared to an early GK Model C.

4. Summary

In this chapter, we have systematically highlighted three state-of-the-art hypofractionated SRS modalities in intracranial applications. With rapid maturing in technology and growing integration of hardware and software in the realm of hypofractionated brain SRS, clinical applications and consensus guidelines are emerging. Both international and national regional societies such as the international stereotactic radiosurgery society (ISRS) and American Association of Physicists in Medicine (AAPM) have initiated joint effort toward developing clinical practice and consensus guidelines. From the physical point of view, future trends in the field will continue to move toward significant enhancements in the areas of (1) imaging guidance, (2) online treatment adaption, and (3) biological tissue effect quantifications for hypofractionated radiosurgery of large and/or complex brain lesions.

Author details

Dilini Pinnaduwage[1], Peng Dong[2] and Lijun Ma[3*]

*Address all correspondence to: lijun.ma@ucsf.edu

1 Department of Radiation Oncology, The University of Arizona School of Medicine/St. Joseph's Hospital Medical Center, Phoenix, AZ, USA

2 Department of Radiation Oncology, Stanford University, Stanford, CA, USA

3 Department of Radiation Oncology, University of California San Francisco, San Francisco, CA, USA

References

[1] Leksell L. 1951. The stereotaxic method and radiosurgery of the brain. *Acta Chir Scand* 102: 316–9.

[2] Wu A, Lindner G, Maitz A H, Kalend A M, Lunsford L D, Flickinger J C and Bloomer W D. 1990. Physics of Gamma Knife approach on convergent beams in stereotactic radiosurgery. *Int J Radiat Oncol Biol Phys* 18: 941–9.

[3] Andrews D W, Bednarz G, Evans J J and Downes B. 2006. A review of 3 current radiosurgery systems. *Surg Neurol* 66: 559–64.

[4] Kano H, Sheehan J, Sneed P K, McBride H L, Young B, Duma C, Mathieu D, Seymour Z, McDermott M W, Kondziolka D, Iyer A and Lunsford L D. 2015. Skull base chondrosarcoma radiosurgery: report of the North American Gamma Knife Consortium. *J Neurosurg* 123: 1268–75.

[5] Regis J, Tuleasca C, Resseguier N, Carron R, Donnet A, Gaudart J and Levivier M. 2016. Long-term safety and efficacy of Gamma Knife surgery in classical trigeminal neuralgia: a 497-patient historical cohort study. *J Neurosurg* 124: 1079–87.

[6] Sahgal A, Ma L, Chang E, Shiu A, Larson D A, Laperriere N, Yin F F, Tsao M, Menard C, Basran P S, Letourneau D, Heydarian M, Beachey D, Shukla V, Cusimano M, Hodaie M, Zadeh G, Bernstein M and Schwartz M. 2009. Advances in technology for intracranial stereotactic radiosurgery. *Technol Cancer Res Treat* 8: 271–80.

[7] Sheehan J P, Kano H, Xu Z, Chiang V, Mathieu D, Chao S, Akpinar B, Lee J Y, Yu J B, Hess J, Wu H M, Chung W Y, Pierce J, Missios S, Kondziolka D, Alonso-Basanta M, Barnett G H and Lunsford L D. 2015a. Gamma Knife radiosurgery for facial nerve schwannomas: a multicenter study. *J Neurosurg* 123: 387–94.

[8] Sheehan J P, Starke R M, Kano H, Barnett G H, Mathieu D, Chiang V, Yu J B, Hess J, McBride H L, Honea N, Nakaji P, Lee J Y, Rahmathulla G, Evanoff W A, Alonso-Basanta M and Lunsford L D. 2015b. Gamma Knife radiosurgery for posterior fossa meningiomas: a multicenter study. *J Neurosurg* 122: 1479–89.

[9] Snell M, Bova F, Larson D, Leavitt D, Lutz W, Podgorsak E and Wu A. 1995. *Stereotactic Radiosurgery, Report of TG42*. Wisconsin: Medical Physics Publishing.

[10] Grandhi R, Kondziolka D, Panczykowski D, Monaco E A, 3rd, Kano H, Niranjan A, Flickinger J C and Lunsford L D. 2012. Stereotactic radiosurgery using the Leksell Gamma Knife Perfexion unit in the management of patients with 10 or more brain metastases. *J Neurosurg* 117: 237–45.

[11] Lindquist C and Paddick I. 2007. The Leksell Gamma Knife Perfexion and comparisons with its predecessors. *Neurosurgery* 61: 130–40; discussion 40-1.

[12] Ma L, Verhey L, Chuang C, Descovich M, Smith V, Huang K, McDermott M and Sneed P. 2008. Effect of composite sector collimation on average dose fall-off for Gamma Knife Perfexion. *J Neurosurg* 109(Suppl): 15–20.

[13] Regis J, Tamura M, Guillot C, Yomo S, Muraciolle X, Nagaje M, Arka Y and Porcheron D. 2009. Radiosurgery with the world's first fully robotized Leksell Gamma Knife PerfeXion in clinical use: a 200-patient prospective, randomized, controlled comparison with the Gamma Knife 4C. *Neurosurgery* 64: 346–55; discussion 55-6.

[14] Al-Omair A, Soliman H, Xu W, Karotki A, Mainprize T, Phan N, Das S, Keith J, Yeung R, Perry J, Tsao M and Sahgal A. 2013. Hypofractionated stereotactic radiotherapy in five daily fractions for post-operative surgical cavities in brain metastases patients with and without prior whole brain radiation. *Technol Cancer Res Treat.* ***12****(6): 493–499*

[15] Devriendt D, De Smedt F, Glineur R and Massager N. 2015. Five-fraction Gamma Knife radiosurgery using the extend relocatable system for benign neoplasms close to optic pathways. *Pract Radiat Oncol* 5: e119–25.

[16] Ma L, Pinnaduwage D, McDermott M and Sneed P K. 2014c. Whole-procedural radiological accuracy for delivering multi-session Gamma Knife radiosurgery with a relocatable frame system. *Technol Cancer Res Treat* 13: 403–8.

[17] Schlesinger D, Xu Z, Taylor F, Yen C P and Sheehan J. 2012. Interfraction and intra-fraction performance of the Gamma Knife extend system for patient positioning and immobilization. *J Neurosurg* 117(Suppl): 217–24.

[18] Ma L, Chiu J, Hoye J, McGuiness C and Perez-Andujar A. 2014a. Quality assurance of stereotactic alignment and patient positioning mechanical accuracy for robotized Gamma Knife radiosurgery. *Phys Med Biol* 59: N221–6.

[19] Paddick I. 2000. A simple scoring ratio to index the conformity of radiosurgical treatment plans. Technical note. *J Neurosurg* 93(Suppl. 3): 219–22.

[20] Paddick I and Lippitz B. 2006. A simple dose gradient measurement tool to complement the conformity index. *J Neurosurg* 105(Suppl): 194–201.

[21] Ma L, Sahgal A, Descovich M, Cho Y B, Chuang C, Huang K, Laperriere N J, Shrieve D C and Larson D A. 2010. Equivalence in dose fall-off for isocentric and nonisocentric intracranial treatment modalities and its impact on dose fractionation schemes. *I J Radiat Oncol, Biol, Phys* 76: 943–8.

[22] Thomas E M, Popple R A, Wu X, Clark G M, Markert J M, Guthrie B L, Yuan Y, Dobelbower M C, Spencer S A and Fiveash J B. 2014. Comparison of plan quality and delivery time between volumetric arc therapy (RapidArc) and Gamma Knife radiosurgery for multiple cranial metastases. *Neurosurgery* 75: 409–17; discussion 17-8.

[23] Ma L, Nichol A, Hossain S, Wang B, Petti P, Vellani R, Higby C, Ahmad S, Barani I, Shrieve D C, Larson D A and Sahgal A. 2014b. Variable dose interplay effects across

radiosurgical apparatus in treating multiple brain metastases. *Int J Comput Assist Radiol Surg*. 9(6): 1079–86

[24] Ma L, Petti P, Wang B, Descovich M, Chuang C, Barani I J, Kunwar S, Shrieve D C, Sahgal A and Larson D A. 2011. Apparatus dependence of normal brain tissue dose in stereotactic radiosurgery for multiple brain metastases. *J Neurosurg* 114: 1580–4.

[25] Ma L, Xia P, Verhey L J and Boyer A L. 1999. A dosimetric comparison of fan-beam intensity modulated radiotherapy with Gamma Knife stereotactic radiosurgery for treating intermediate intracranial lesions. *Int J Radiat Oncol Biol Phys* 45: 1325–30.

[26] Luan S, Swanson N, Chen Z and Ma L. 2009. Dynamic Gamma Knife radiosurgery. *Phys Med Biol* 54: 1579–91.

[27] Ma L, Mason E, Sneed P K, McDermott M, Polishchuk A, Larson D A and Sahgal A. 2015. Clinical realization of sector beam intensity modulation for Gamma Knife radiosurgery: a pilot treatment planning study. *Int J Radiat Oncol Biol Phys* 91: 661–8.

[28] Adler JR.(1993) Frameless Radiosurgery. In Stereotactic Surgery and Radiosurgery, ed. AAF De Salles and SJ Goetsch, 237–48. Madison: Medical Physics Publishing.

[29] Adler JR, Cox RS. 1996. *Preliminary Experience with CyberKnife – Radiosurgery*. Basel: S. Karger; pp. 112–38.

[30] Kilby W, Dooley J R, Kuduvalli G, Sayeh S and Maurer C R, Jr. 2010. The CyberKnife robotic radiosurgery system in 2010. *Technol Cancer Res Treat* 9: 433–52.

[31] Echner G G, Kilby W, Lee M, Earnst E, Sayeh S, Schlaefer A, Rhein B, Dooley J R, Lang C, Blanck O, Lessard E, Maurer C R, Jr. and Schlegel W. 2009. The design, physical properties and clinical utility of an iris collimator for robotic radiosurgery. *Phys Med Biol* 54: 5359–80.

[32] Accuray Inc. 2013 *CyberKnife M6 Series Technical Specifications*. Madison, WI: Accuray.

[33] Pinnaduwage DS, Descovich M and Ma L. 2014. Treatment planning, intrafractional tracking and delivery: CyberKnife-based stereotactic body radiation therapy. *Stereotactic Body Radiat Therapy Spinal Metastasis*, ed. SL Simon, A Sahgal, BS The, PC Gerszten and EL Chang, 57–75. UK: Future Science Group.

[34] Adler J R, Jr., Murphy M J, Chang S D and Hancock S L. 1999. Image-guided robotic radiosurgery. *Neurosurgery* 44: 1299–306; discussion 306-7.

[35] Francescon P, Kilby W, Satariano N and Cora S. 2012. Monte Carlo simulated correction factors for machine specific reference field dose calibration and output factor measurement using fixed and iris collimators on the CyberKnife system. *Phys Med Biol* 57: 3741–58.

[36] Pantelis E, Moutsatsos A, Zourari K, Petrokokkinos L, Sakelliou L, Kilby W, Antypas C, Papagiannis P, Karaiskos P, Georgiou E and Seimenis I. 2012. On the output factor measurements of the CyberKnife iris collimator small fields: experimental determina-

tion of the k(Q(clin),Q(msr)) (f(clin),f(msr)) correction factors for microchamber and diode detectors. *Med Phys* 39: 4875–85.

[37] Schlaefer A and Schweikard A. 2008. Stepwise multi-criteria optimization for robotic radiosurgery. *Med Phys* 35: 2094–103.

[38] Wilcox E E, Daskalov G M, Lincoln H, Shumway R C, Kaplan B M and Colasanto J M. 2010. Comparison of planned dose distributions calculated by Monte Carlo and Ray-Trace algorithms for the treatment of lung tumors with cyberknife: a preliminary study in 33 patients. *Int J Radiat Oncol Biol Phys* 77: 277–84.

[39] Wilcox E E, Daskalov G M and Lincoln H. 2011. Stereotactic radiosurgery-radiotherapy: Should Monte Carlo treatment planning be used for all sites? *Pract Radiat Oncol* 1: 251–60.

[40] Benedict S H, Yenice K M, Followill D, Galvin J M, Hinson W, Kavanagh B, Keall P, Lovelock M, Meeks S, Papiez L, Purdie T, Sadagopan R, Schell M C, Salter B, Schlesinger D J, Shiu A S, Solberg T, Song D Y, Stieber V, Timmerman R, Tome W A, Verellen D, Wang L and Yin F F. 2010. Stereotactic body radiation therapy: the report of AAPM Task Group 101. *Med Phys* 37: 4078–101.

[41] Jeong W J, Park J H, Lee E J, Kim J H, Kim C J and Cho Y H. 2015. Efficacy and safety of fractionated stereotactic radiosurgery for large brain metastases. *J Korean Neurosurg Soc* 58: 217–24.

[42] Inoue H K, Sato H, Seto K, Torikai K, Suzuki Y, Saitoh J, Noda S E and Nakano T. 2014. Five-fraction CyberKnife radiotherapy for large brain metastases in critical areas: impact on the surrounding brain volumes circumscribed with a single dose equivalent of 14 Gy (V14) to avoid radiation necrosis. *J Radiat Res* 55: 334–42.

[43] Okamoto H, Hamada M, Sakamoto, Wakita A, Nakamura S, Kato T, Abe Y, Takahashi K, Igaki H and Itami J. 2016. Log-file analysis of accuracy of beam localization for brain tumor treatment by CyberKnife. *Prac Radiat Oncol* In press.

[44] McGuinness C M, Gottschalk A R, Lessard E, Nakamura J L, Pinnaduwage D, Pouliot J, Sims C and Descovich M. 2015. Investigating the clinical advantages of a robotic linac equipped with a multileaf collimator in the treatment of brain and prostate cancer patients. *J Appl Clin Med Phys* 16: 5502.

[45] Lutz W, Winston K R and Maleki N. 1988. A system for stereotactic radiosurgery with a linear accelerator. *Int J Radiat Oncol Biol Phys* 14: 373–81.

[46] Winston K R and Lutz W. 1988. Linear accelerator as a neurosurgical tool for stereotactic radiosurgery. *Neurosurgery* 22: 454–64.

[47] Narayanasamy G, Saenz D, Cruz W, Ha C S, Papanikolaou N and Stathakis S. 2016. Commissioning an Elekta Versa HD linear accelerator. *J Appl Clin Med Phys* 17: 5799.

[48] Thomas E M, Popple R A, Prendergast B M, Clark G M, Dobelbower M C and Fiveash J B. 2013. Effects of flattening filter-free and volumetric-modulated arc therapy delivery on treatment efficiency. *J Appl Clin Med Phys* 14: 4328.

[49] Tryggestad E, Christian M, Ford E, Kut C, Le Y, Sanguineti G, Song D Y and Kleinberg L. 2011. Inter- and intrafraction patient positioning uncertainties for intracranial radiotherapy: a study of four frameless, thermoplastic mask-based immobilization strategies using daily cone-beam CT. *Int J Radiat Oncol Biol Phys* 80: 281–90.

[50] Schmidhalter D, Fix M K, Wyss M, Schaer N, Munro P, Scheib S, Kunz P and Manser P. 2013. Evaluation of a new six degrees of freedom couch for radiation therapy. *Med Phys* 40: 111710.

[51] Guckenberger M, Meyer J, Wilbert J, Baier K, Sauer O and Flentje M. 2007. Precision of image-guided radiotherapy (IGRT) in six degrees of freedom and limitations in clinical practice. *Strahlenther Onkol* 183: 307–13.

[52] Mayo C S, Ding L, Addesa A, Kadish S, Fitzgerald T J and Moser R. 2010. Initial experience with volumetric IMRT (RapidArc) for intracranial stereotactic radiosurgery. *Int J Radiat Oncol Biol Phys* 78: 1457–66.